should be 356

NOT
7560 mg 90

RENAL
PHYSIOLOGY

RENAL
PHYSIOLOGY

ARTHUR J. VANDER, M.D.

Professor of Physiology
University of Michigan

McGRAW-HILL BOOK COMPANY
A Blakiston Publication
New York   St. Louis   San Francisco   Auckland   Düsseldorf
Johannesburg   Kuala Lumpur   London   Mexico   Montreal   New Delhi
Panama   Paris   São Paulo   Singapore   Sydney   Tokyo   Toronto

NOTICE

Medicine is an ever-changing science. As new research and clinical experience broaden our knowledge, changes in treatment and drug therapy are required. The editors and the publisher of this work have made every effort to ensure that the drug dosage schedules herein are accurate and in accord with the standards accepted at the time of publication. The reader is advised, however, to check the product information sheet included in the package of each drug he plans to administer to be certain that changes have not been made in the recommended dose or in the contraindications for administration. This recommendation is of particular importance in regard to new or infrequently used drugs.

RENAL PHYSIOLOGY

3 4 5 6 7 8 9 0   KPKP   7 9 8 7

This book was set in Times Roman by Progressive Typographers.
The editors were J. Dereck Jeffers and Carol First;
the cover was designed by Nicholas Krenitsky;
the production supervisor was Judi Frey.
New drawings were done by Eric G. Hieber Associates Inc.
Kingsport Press, Inc., was printer and binder.

Library of Congress Cataloging in Publication Data

Vander, Arthur J   date
 Renal physiology.

 "A Blakiston publication."
 Bibliography: p.
 1. Kidneys. I. Title. [DNLM: 1. Kidney--
Physiology.   WJ300 V229r]
QP249.V36   612'.463   75-1302
ISBN 0-07-066957-0

CONTENTS

PREFACE

This book is my attempt to identify the essential core content of renal physiology appropriate for medical students and to present it in a way which permits the student to master the material independently, i.e., with no (or very few) accompanying lectures by the instructor. The book's ability to serve as the sole source of information for most students has been tested at the University of Michigan for the past 3 years and has been well substantiated in terms of student examination performance and enthusiasm.

My selection of this core material is made explicit in a comprehensive list of behavioral objectives, which tell the student specifically what I believe he should know and be able to do by the book's completion. Obviously, no two instructors would come up with exactly the same core material, but it is a simple matter for the instructor to give his students a supplementary list of goals to be added or deleted. The information required to achieve any additional goals not covered in the book would, of course, have to be provided by other reading assignments or lectures.

However, my belief, based on consultations with other physiologists and clinicians, is that these discrepancies are likely to be few. Of much greater importance is the fact that the behavioral goals (in essence, the content of the book) are explicitly defined so that any such differences are easily determined. This also makes the book quite usable for students in other health sciences whose required core of information might differ from that of medical students.

In addition to the comprehensive objectives, I have included a large number of study questions with annotated answers. Unlike the lists of objectives, the study questions are neither systematic nor comprehensive in their coverage. Rather, they generally deal with areas I have found usually difficult for students and give them practice and additional feedback.

I advise the student to go through the book one chapter at a time. Some students profit by using the objectives to guide their readings as they proceed through a chapter. In any case, at the end of each chapter go over the objectives in detail and the study questions (at the back of the book) relevant to that chapter. They provide you with the means for determining whether you have mastered the material and for identifying those specific areas which require more work.

I should like to point out several characteristics of the book common to most texts but particularly common in this type of book. I have rarely included the original research upon which this core of knowledge rests, nor have I been able to explore the fascinating controversies in virtually every area. Therefore, the Suggested Readings at the back of the book are of considerable importance for the student who wishes to pursue any subject in greater depth. They are almost all review articles, and their bibliographies provide an entry into the original research literature. The question of how to handle controversy in such a book is a particularly perplexing one. I have tried to present various views (frequently in footnotes) in areas where the evidence is closely balanced, but I have often simply had to ignore an opposing view. Obviously, such decisions are always arbitrary, to a large degree, and I can only apologize, in advance, to those of my colleagues who feel I have slighted their work.

I sincerely request students and instructors to inform me of factual errors and of portions which are unclearly written. In addition, I would greatly appreciate your views about which goals and objectives you feel should be added, removed, or altered in emphasis.

Finally, I again thank Helen Mysyk for her splendid typing.

Arthur J. Vander

RENAL
PHYSIOLOGY

Chapter 1

Function and Structure of the Kidneys

OBJECTIVES

The student lists the basic functions of the kidney.
1 Regulation of ionic composition of extracellular fluid
2 Excretion of metabolic end products
3 Secretion of renin and renal erythropoietic factor
4 Activation of vitamin D
5 Gluconeogenesis during prolonged fasting

The student defines important anatomical structures and knows their interrelationships.
   Nephron, glomerulus, tubule, Bowman's capsule, proximal and distal tubules, juxtaglomerular apparatus, loop of Henle, afferent and efferent arterioles, vasa recta, medulla, cortex, collecting ducts, superficial cortex and nephrons, juxtamedullary cortex and nephrons, renal pelvis

FUNCTION

A cell's function depends not only upon receiving a continuous supply of nutrients and eliminating its metabolic end products but also upon the

1

existence of stable physicochemical conditions in the extracellular fluid bathing it, Claude Bernard's "internal environment." Maintenance of this stability is the primary function of the kidneys.

Since the extracellular fluid occupies an intermediate position between the external environment and the cells, the concentration of any substance within it can be altered by exchange in either direction. Exchanges with cells are called *internal exchanges.* For example, a decrease in extracellular potassium concentration is followed by a counteracting movement of potassium out of cells into the extracellular fluid. Each type of ion is stored in cells or in bone in significant amounts, which can be partially depleted or expanded without damage to the storage site. But these stores are limited, and in the long run any deficit or excess of total body water or total body electrolyte must be compensated by exchanges with the external environment, i.e., by changes in intake or output.

A substance appears in the body either as a result of ingestion or as a product of metabolism. Conversely, a substance can be excreted from the body or consumed in a metabolic reaction. Therefore, if the quantity of any substance in the body is to be maintained at a constant level over a period of time, the total amounts ingested and produced must equal the total amounts excreted and consumed. This is a general statement of the *balance concept.* For water and hydrogen ion all four possible pathways apply. However, balance is simpler for the mineral electrolytes. Since they are neither synthesized nor consumed by cells, their total body balance reflects only ingestion versus excretion.

As an example, let us describe the balance for total body water (Table 1). It should be recognized that these are average values, which are subject to considerable variation. The two sources of body water are metabolically produced water, resulting largely from the oxidation of carbohydrates, and ingested water, obtained from liquids and so-called solid food (a rare steak is approximately 70 percent water).

Table 1   Normal Routes of Water Gain and Loss in Adults

Route	ml/day
Intake	
Drunk	1,200
In food	1,000
Metabolically produced	350
Total	2,550
Output	
Insensible loss (skin and lungs)	900
Sweat	50
In feces	100
Urine	1,500
Total	2,550

There are four sites from which water is lost to the external environment: skin, lungs, gastrointestinal tract, and kidneys. The loss of water by evaporation from the cells of the skin and the lining of respiratory passageways is a continuous process, often referred to as *insensible loss* because the person is unaware of its occurrence. Additional water can be made available for evaporation from the skin by the production of sweat. The normal gastrointestinal loss of water (in feces) is quite small but can be severe in vomiting or diarrhea.

Under normal conditions, as can be seen from the table, water loss exactly equals water gain, and no net change of body water occurs. This is obviously no accident but the result of precise regulatory mechanisms. The question then is: Which processes involved in water balance are controlled to make the gains and losses balance? The answer, as we shall see, is voluntary intake (*thirst*) and urinary loss. This does not mean that none of the other processes is controlled, but it does mean their control is not primarily oriented toward water balance. Carbohydrate catabolism, the major source of water from oxidation, is controlled by mechanisms directed toward regulation of energy balance. Sweat production is controlled by mechanisms directed toward temperature regulation. Insensible loss in man is truly uncontrolled. Fecal water loss is generally unchanging and is normally quite small.

The mechanism of thirst is certainly of great importance, since body deficits of water, regardless of cause, must be made up by ingestion of water. But it is also true that our fluid intake is often influenced more by habit and by sociological factors than by the need to regulate body water. The control of urinary water loss is the major automatic mechanism by which body water is regulated.

By similar analyses, we find that the body balances of most of the ions determining the properties of the extracellular fluid are regulated primarily by the kidneys. To appreciate the importance of these kidney regulations one need only make a partial list of the more important simple inorganic substances which constitute the internal environment and which are regulated in large part by the kidney: water, sodium, potassium, chloride, calcium, magnesium, sulfate, phosphate, and hydrogen ion. Indeed, the extraordinary number of substances which the kidney regulates and the precision with which these processes normally occur accounted for the kidney's being the last stronghold of the nineteenth century vitalists, who simply would not believe that the laws of physics and chemistry could fully explain renal function. By what mechanism does urine flow rapidly increase when a person ingests several glasses of liquid? How is it that the patient on an extremely low salt intake and the person who eats a great deal of salt both urinate precisely the amounts of salt required to maintain their sodium balance? What mechanisms decrease the urinary calcium excretion of children deprived of milk?

This regulatory role is obviously quite different from the popular conception of the kidneys as glorified garbage-disposal units which rid the body of assorted wastes and poisons. It is true that several of the complex chemical reactions which occur within cells result ultimately in end products that must be eliminated. These end products are often called waste products because they serve no known biological function in man. For example, the catabolism of protein produces approximately 50 gm of urea per day. Other end products produced in relatively large quantities are uric acid (from nucleic acids), creatinine (from muscle creatine), the end products of hemoglobin breakdown, and the metabolites of various hormones. There are many others, not all of which have been completely identified. Most of these substances are eliminated from the body as rapidly as they are produced, primarily by way of the kidneys. Some of these end products, e.g., urea, are relatively harmless, although the accumulation of others within the body during periods of renal malfunction accounts for some of the disordered body functions in the patient suffering from severe kidney disease. We still are not sure which of the problems occurring in renal disease are due to these "toxins" and which are due to disordered water-and-electrolyte metabolism.

The kidneys have another excretory function, which is presently assuming increasing importance, namely, the elimination from the body of foreign chemicals, such as drugs, pesticides, and food additives, and their metabolites.

In addition to these regulatory and excretory tasks, the kidneys perform several other functions:

1   They serve as important endocrine glands secreting *renin* and *renal erythropoietic factor*. The former hormone will be discussed in detail subsequently; the latter is an important component of the erythropoietin system, a hormonal system which controls erythrocyte production.

2   They activate vitamin D by altering its molecular structure.

3   During prolonged fasting, they synthesize glucose and release it into the blood. Thus, like the liver, they are a gluconeogenic organ.

STRUCTURE OF THE KIDNEYS AND URINARY SYSTEM

The kidneys are paired organs which lie outside the peritoneal cavity in the back of the abdominal wall, one on each side of the vertebral column. In man, each kidney is composed of approximately 1 million tiny units. One such unit, or *nephron,* is shown in Fig. 1. The nephron consists of a vascular component called the *glomerulus* and a *tubular component*. The mechanisms by which the kidneys perform their functions depend on the relationships between these two components.

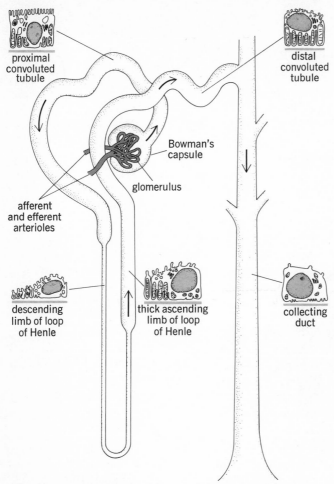

proximal
convoluted
tubule

distal
convoluted
tubule

Bowman's
capsule

glomerulus

afferent
and efferent
arterioles

descending
limb of loop
of Henle

thick ascending
limb of loop
of Henle

collecting
duct

Figure 1   Relationships of component parts of the nephron. [*Drawings of fine structure adapted from T. Rhodin,* Int. Rev. Cytol., **7:485** *(1958).*]

Throughout its course, the tubule is composed of a single layer of epithelial cells, which differ in structure and function from portion to portion, as will be described below. It originates as a balloonlike, blind-ended sac, known as *Bowman's capsule,* which is lined with thin epithelial cells. On one side, Bowman's capsule is intimately associated with the glomerulus; on the other, it opens into the first portion of the tubule, which is highly coiled and is known as the *proximal convoluted tubule.* The next portion of the tubule is a sharp hairpinlike loop, called the *loop of Henle.* The tubule once more becomes coiled (the *distal convoluted tubule*) and finally runs a straight course as the *collecting duct.* From the glomerulus to the beginning of the collecting duct, each of the 1 million

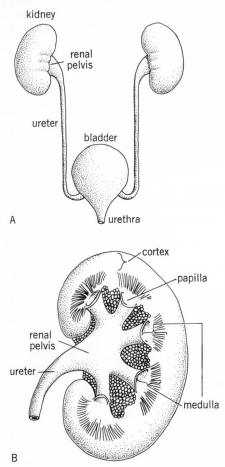

Figure 2 A. The urinary system. The urine, formed by the kidney, collects in the renal pelvis and then flows through the ureter into the bladder, from which it is eliminated via the urethra. B. Section of a human kidney. Half the kidney has been sliced away. Note that the structure shows regional differences. The outer portion (cortex), which has a granular appearance, contains all the glomeruli. The collecting ducts form a large portion of the inner kidney (medulla), giving it a striped, pyramidlike appearance, and drain into the renal pelvis. The papilla is the inner portion of the medulla. (*From A. J. Vander et al., "Human Physiology,"* © *1970 by McGraw-Hill, Inc. Used with permission of McGraw-Hill Book Company.*)

tubules is completely separate from its neighbors. The tiny collecting ducts from separate tubules join to form larger ducts, which in turn join to form even larger ducts, which finally empty into a large central cavity, the *renal pelvis,* at the base of each kidney (Fig. 2). The renal pelvis is continuous with the *ureter,* which empties into the *urinary bladder,* where urine is temporarily stored and from which it is intermittently eliminated. The urine is not altered after it leaves the collecting ducts.

From the renal pelvis on, the remainder of the urinary system simply serves as plumbing.

To return to the other component of the nephron: What is the origin and nature of the glomerulus? Blood enters the kidney via the renal artery, which then divides into progressively smaller branches. Each of the smallest arteries gives off, at right angles to itself, a series of *afferent arterioles* (Fig. 3), each of which leads to a compact tuft of capillaries. This tuft of capillaries is the glomerulus, which protrudes into Bowman's capsule, essentially floating in the fluid within the capsule (Fig. 4). The functional significance of this anatomical arrangement is that blood in the glomerulus is separated from the fluid within Bowman's capsule only by the capillary membranes. This thin barrier permits the filtration of fluid from the capillaries into Bowman's capsule.

In virtually all other organs capillaries recombine to form the beginnings of the venous system. The glomerular capillaries instead recombine to form another set of arterioles, called the *efferent arterioles*. Thus, blood leaves the glomerulus through an arteriole which soon subdivides

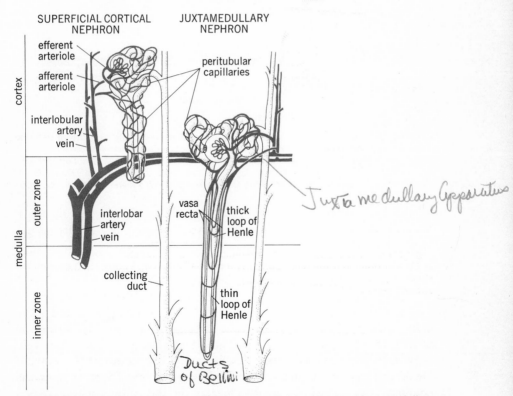

Figure 3 Comparison of the blood supplies of superficial cortical and juxtamedullary nephrons. (*Redrawn from R. F. Pitts, "Physiology of the Kidney and Body Fluids," 3d ed., Year Book, Chicago, 1974.*)

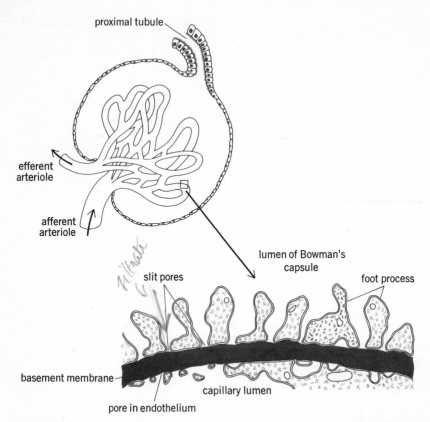

Figure 4   Anatomy of the glomerulus (See page 14 for description). Bottom drawing shows the glomerular membrane: tubular epithelium (only foot processes are shown), basement membrane, and capillary endothelium. [*Adapted from C. Rouiller and A. F. Muller (eds.), "The Kidney," Academic, New York, 1969, and H. Valtin "Renal Function," Little, Brown, Boston, 1973. Fine structure redrawn from an electron micrograph by C. C. Tisher.*]

into a second set of capillaries (Fig. 3). These *peritubular capillaries* are profusely distributed to, and intimately associated with, all the remaining portions of the tubule. They rejoin to form the venous channels by which blood ultimately leaves the kidney.

There are important regional differences in the location of the various tubular and vascular components. As shown in Figs. 2 and 3, the kidney can be divided into an outer portion, called the *cortex*, and an inner portion, called the *medulla*. The cortex contains all the glomeruli, proximal and distal convoluted tubules, and first portions of the loops of Henle and collecting ducts. In man, approximately 85 percent of the nephrons originate in glomeruli located in the outer, or *superficial*, cortex and have relatively short loops of Henle, which extend only into the outer medulla. The remaining 15 percent originate in glomeruli located in the innermost, or *juxtamedullary,* cortex (i.e., "cortex just adjacent to the medulla"). These so-called *juxtamedullary nephrons,* in contrast to the *superficial nephrons,* have long loops which extend deep into the medulla, where they run parallel to the collecting ducts. The vascular structure supplying the juxtamedullary nephrons also differs in that its efferent arterioles drain not only into the usual peritubular-capillary network of the cortex but also into thin hairpin-loop vessels (*vasa recta*), which run parallel to the loops of Henle and collecting ducts in the medulla. This arrangement has considerable significance for renal function, as will be described later.

One last anatomical feature should be pointed out. Note that, as the loop ascends into the cortex to become the distal tubule, the tubule contacts the arterioles supplying its nephron of origin. This area of contact is marked by unique structural changes in both the arterioles and tubules and is known as the *juxtaglomerular apparatus*. Its structure and function will also be discussed later on.

Study question: **1**

Chapter 2

Basic Renal Processes

OBJECTIVES

The student knows the basic principles of renal physiology.
1 Lists and defines the three renal processes: glomerular filtration, tubular reabsorption, tubular secretion
2 Describes the routes for blood and fluid movements within the kidneys
3 Describes the anatomy of the glomerular capillaries
4 Describes the chemical characteristics of the glomerular filtrate
5 States the formula for the determinants of glomerular net filtration pressure and the normal values for each determinant
6 Describes the method and formula used for measurement of GFR
7 Distinguishes between active and passive transport
8 Defines transepithelial transport
9 Distinguishes between the mechanisms underlying glomerular filtration, on the one hand, and tubular reabsorption and secretion, on the other
10 Defines the concept of T_m (either reabsorptive or secretory); given appropriate data, calculates T_m; defines splay and describes the mechanism for it

11 Compares the transport mechanisms for glucose and phosphate
12 States the significance of a T_m being much higher than the usual filtered mass of the substance
13 Describes the renal handling of protein
14 Describes the renal handling of urea

Urine formation begins with the filtration of essentially protein-free plasma through the glomerular capillaries into Bowman's capsule. The final urine which enters the renal pelvis is quite different from the *glomerular filtrate* because, as the filtered fluid flows from Bowman's capsule through the remaining portions of the tubule, its composition is altered. This change occurs by two general processes: tubular reabsorption and tubular secretion. The tubule is at all points intimately associated with the peritubular capillaries, a relationship that permits transfer of materials between the peritubular plasma and the inside of the tubule, or *tubular lumen*. When the direction of transfer is from tubular lumen to peritubular-capillary plasma, the process is called *tubular reabsorption*. Movement in the opposite direction, i.e., from peritubular plasma to tubular lumen, is called *tubular secretion*. This term must not be confused with excretion. To say that a substance has been excreted is to say that it appears in the final urine. These relationships are illustrated in Fig. 5.

The most common relationships between these basic renal processes — glomerular filtration, tubular reabsorption, and tubular secretion — are shown in Fig. 6. Plasma containing substances X, Y, and Z enters the glomerular capillaries. A certain quantity of protein-free plasma containing these substances is filtered into Bowman's capsule, enters the proximal tubule, and begins its flow through the rest of the tubule. The remainder of the plasma, also containing X, Y, and Z, leaves the glomerular capillaries via an efferent arteriole and enters the peritubular capillaries. The cells composing the tubular epithelium can transport X (not Y or Z) from the peritubular plasma into the tubular lumen, but not in the opposite direction. By this combination of filtration and tubular secretion all the plasma which originally entered the renal artery is cleared of substance X, which leaves the body via the urine, thus reducing the amount of X remaining in the body. If the tubule were incapable of reabsorption, the Y and Z originally filtered at the glomerulus would also leave the body via the urine, but the tubule can transport Y and Z from the tubular lumen back into the peritubular plasma. The amount of reabsorption of Y is small, so most of the filtered material does escape from the body. But for Z the reabsorptive mechanism is so powerful that virtually all the filtered material is transported back into the plasma, which flows through the renal vein back into the vena cava. Therefore no Z is lost from the body. Hence the processes of filtration

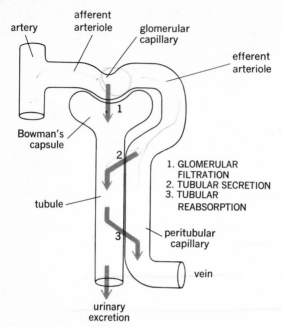

Figure 5   The three basic components of renal function. (*From A. J. Vander et al., "Human Physiology,"* © *1970 by McGraw-Hill, Inc. Used with permission of McGraw-Hill Book Company.*)

and reabsorption have canceled out each other, and the net result is as though Z had never entered the kidney at all.

The kidney works only on plasma; the erythrocytes supply oxygen to the kidney but serve no other function in urine formation. Each substance in plasma is handled in a characteristic manner by the nephron, i.e., by a particular combination of filtration, reabsorption, and secretion. (Tubular synthesis with subsequent release of the synthesized products into either the blood or the tubular lumen might well be listed as a fourth basic renal process. For example, we shall see that the tubular cells synthesize ammonia.) The critical point is that *the rates at which the relevant basic processes proceed for many of these substances are subject to physiological control.* What is the effect, for example, if the filtered mass of Y is increased or its reabsorption rate decreased? Either change causes more Y to be lost from the body via the urine. By triggering such changes in filtration or reabsorption whenever the plasma concentration of Y rises above normal, homeostatic mechanisms regulate plasma Y.

In summary, one can study the normal renal handling of any given substance by asking a series of questions:

1   To what degree is the substance filtered at the glomerulus?
2   Is it reabsorbed?

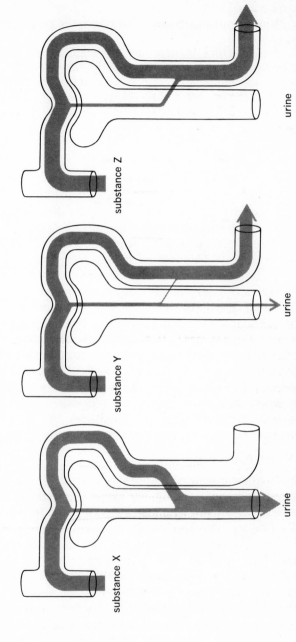

Figure 6 Renal manipulation of three substances, X, Y, and Z. X is filtered, and a fraction is then reabsorbed. Z is filtered but is completely reabsorbed. Y is filtered and secreted but not reabsorbed. (*From A. J. Vander et al., "Human Physiology."* © *1970 by McGraw-Hill, Inc. Used with permission of McGraw-Hill Book Company.*)

3 Is it secreted?

4 What are the mechanisms by which the reabsorption or secretion is achieved?

5 What factors homeostatically regulate the quantities filtered, reabsorbed, or secreted; i.e., what are the reflexes by which renal excretion of the substance is altered so as to maintain stable body balance?

6 What factors other than renal disease can perturb body balance of the substance by causing the kidneys to filter, reabsorb, or secrete too much or too little of the substance?

GLOMERULAR FILTRATION

The capillaries of the body are freely permeable to water and to *crystalloids,* which are solutes of small molecular dimensions. They are relatively impermeable to large molecules, or *colloids,* the most important of which are the plasma proteins. The glomerulus behaves qualitatively like any other capillary. This may seem surprising since the glomerular barrier is structurally different from other capillaries in that it is composed of three layers (Fig. 4): capillary endothelium, basement membrane, and a single-celled layer of epithelial cells. These epithelial cells (podocytes) have an unusual octopuslike structure in that they have a large number of extensions, or foot processes, which rest on the basement membrane. Slits exist between adjacent foot processes and probably constitute the path through which the filtrate, once past the endothelial cells and basement membrane, travels to enter Bowman's capsule. The presence of this epithelial layer may account for certain quantitative differences between the glomerulus and other capillaries.

Composition of the Filtrate

The fluid within Bowman's capsule is essentially protein-free and contains crystalloids in virtually the same concentrations as the plasma does. These facts were established by the work of A. N. Richards and his collaborators, who developed the theoretically simple but technically complicated method of *micropuncture.* The nephrons of amphibians are relatively large and can be seen easily, since they are not packed together into an enclosed organ like the human kidneys. These scientists inserted tiny micropipets into Bowman's capsule and withdrew extremely small quantities of fluid, which they analyzed. They demonstrated that the fluid in Bowman's capsule contains little or no protein and that all crystalloids measured (glucose, hydrogen ion, chloride, potassium, phosphate, urea, creatinine, and uric acid) were present in virtually the same concentrations as they were in the plasma. Actually, the concentrations of the crystalloids in Bowman's capsule are not precisely the same as in plasma because of the difference in protein concentration between these fluids. This effect is very small and may be ignored. More importantly, any crystalloid which is partially bound to protein will have a lower concentration in Bowman's capsule than in the plasma because the protein-bound moiety will not filter. The concentration in Bowman's capsule will equal the *free,* i.e., unbound, concentration in plasma.

Micropuncture has also been used to withdraw fluid from almost all portions of the tubule. Its application to mammals, as well as to amphibians, has provided many of the fundamental facts of renal physiology.

Forces Involved in Filtration

According to Starling's hypothesis, the *net filtration pressure* NFP for any capillary is the algebraic sum of the opposing hydrostatic and colloid osmotic pressures acting across the capillary. This law also applies to the glomerular capillaries:

$$\text{NFP} = \quad (P_{GC} + \pi_{BC}) \quad - \quad (P_{BC} + \pi_{GC})$$
$$\text{Forces inducing filtration} \quad \text{Forces opposing filtration}$$

where P_{GC} = glomerular-capillary hydrostatic pressure
   π_{BC} = colloid osmotic pressure of fluid in Bowman's capsule
   P_{BC} = hydrostatic pressure in Bowman's capsule
   π_{GC} = colloid osmotic pressure in glomerular-capillary plasma

Because there is virtually no protein in Bowman's capsule, π_{BC} may be taken as zero so that the equation becomes

$$\text{NFP} = P_{GC} - P_{BC} - \pi_{GC}$$

The estimated normal values of these forces in man are given in Table 2. Note that their magnitudes at the beginning of the glomerular capillaries differ from their magnitudes at the end of the glomerular capillaries. The changes in magnitudes are caused by two factors: (1) Capillary hydrostatic pressure decreases slightly because of the resistance to flow offered by the capillaries. (2) Colloid osmotic pressure increases because, since the filtrate is essentially protein-free, the filtration process removes water but not protein from the plasma, thereby increasing the protein concentration of the unfiltered plasma remaining in the capillaries. Normally about 20 percent of the plasma water is filtered, accounting for the increase in colloid osmotic pressure from 25 mmHg in the afferent end to 35 mmHg in the efferent end. The latter value for pressure is more than 25/0.8 because the relationship between colloid osmotic pressure and plasma protein concentration is not linear.

Table 2   Estimated Forces Involved in Glomerular Filtration in Man

	mmHg	
Forces	Afferent end of glomerular capillary	Efferent end of glomerular capillary
1. Favoring filtration		
Glomerular capillary hydrostatic pressure P_{GC}	47	45
2. Opposing filtration		
a. Hydrostatic pressure in Bowman's capsule P_{BC}	10	10
b. Colloid osmotic pressure in glomerular capillary π_{GC}	25	35
3. Net filtration pressure $[(1) - (2)]$	12	0

For complex reasons we have not described, colloid osmotic pressure increases more than linearly with protein concentration.

It must be emphasized that the hydrostatic pressures in Table 2 are only *estimates,* since no micropuncture measurements of the true pressures have ever been performed in man. Such measurements have been made in other mammals and are used as the basis for the estimates.

Table 2 reveals that the net filtration pressure is quite small, 12 mmHg at the beginning of the capillary and 0 mmHg at the end. This latter number is quite significant, since it means that no filtration is occurring at all by the end of the capillary. That is, the rise in colloid osmotic pressure resulting from filtration has become high enough to completely counteract the hydrostatic pressure gradient and prevent any further filtration. The figure we would like to have is the *mean net filtration pressure,* i.e., the NFP averaged over the entire capillary length. Clearly, it is somewhere between 12 and 0, but no exact number can be determined, since we do not know how soon NFP becomes 0 along the capillary. It is sufficient to recognize that the normal mean NFP is almost certainly no more than 5 to 6 mmHg. This pressure initiates urine formation by forcing an essentially protein-free filtrate of plasma through the glomerular membranes into Bowman's capsule, and thence down the tubule. In the next section we shall see that the normal rate of formation of glomerular filtrate is 125 ml/min. That a mean net filtration pressure of only 5 to 6 mmHg or less suffices to filter this large quantity of fluid is explainable by the fact that, relative to extrarenal capillaries, the glomerular capillaries occupy a larger surface area per unit of tissue and are many times more permeable to water and crystalloids. It should be reemphasized that the glomerular membranes serve only as a filtration barrier and play no active, i.e., energy-requiring, role. The energy which produces glomerular filtration is the energy transmitted to the blood as hydrostatic pressure when the heart contracts.

Before leaving this topic, we must point out the reason for our use of the term "essentially protein-free" in describing the glomerular filtrate. In reality there is a very small amount of protein in the filtrate. The glomerular membranes are not perfect sieves for protein. Normally, much less than 1 percent of serum albumin and almost no globulin is filtered; the fate of this filtered protein will be described later. Hemoglobin is not normally filtered, because it is totally contained in the erythrocytes. However, when abnormal erythrocyte destruction does cause hemoglobin to appear in the plasma, a significant fraction is filtered. This is also true of muscle myoglobin released as a result of muscle damage. These facts, as well as the data from many other experimental studies, lead to the conclusion that the glomerular-capillary membranes (endothelium, basement membrane, and epithelium) behave as though they were a sieve perforated by 75 to 100 Å pores. However, whether such pores actually exist or whether the functional properties actually reflect a hydrated gel structure of the membrane, instead, remains an unsettled question.

Rate of Filtration

In man, the average volume of fluid filtered from the plasma into Bowman's capsule is 180 liters/day (approximately 45 gal)! The implications of this remarkable fact are extremely important. When we recall that the average total volume of plasma in man is approximately 3 liters, it follows that the entire plasma volume is filtered by the kidneys some 60 times a day. It is, in part, this ability to process such huge volumes of plasma that enables the kidneys to excrete large quantities of waste products and to regulate the constituents of the internal environment so precisely. The second implication concerns the magnitude of the reabsorptive process. The average person excretes between 1 and 2 liters of urine per day. Since 180 liters of fluid are filtered, approximately 99 percent of the filtered water must have been reabsorbed into the peritubular capillaries, the remaining 1 percent escaping from the body as urinary water.

What factors directly determine the magnitude of the glomerular filtration rate? The answer is: simply the algebraic sum of the Starling forces summarized in Table 2. Accordingly, any change either in the hydrostatic pressures within the glomerular capillaries or Bowman's capsule or in the colloid osmotic pressure of the plasma can alter the net filtration pressure. For example, occlusion of the ureter will, by damming the urine, cause a rise in intratubular pressure all the way back to Bowman's capsule. The result is a decreased net filtration pressure and a reduced glomerular filtration rate. Another example: Loss of a significant quantity of protein-free extracellular fluid, such as occurs during sweating or diarrhea, increases the plasma colloid osmotic pressure,

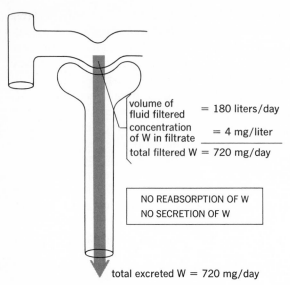

volume of
fluid filtered   = 180 liters/day

concentration
of W in filtrate   = 4 mg/liter

total filtered W = 720 mg/day

NO REABSORPTION OF W
NO SECRETION OF W

total excreted W = 720 mg/day

Figure 7   The measurement of glomerular filtration. W is filtered but is neither reabsorbed nor secreted. (*From A. J. Vander et al., "Human Physiology," © 1970 by
McGraw-Hill, Inc. Used with permission of McGraw-Hill Book Company.*)

thereby reducing net filtration pressure and glomerular filtration rate.
These examples illustrate how changes either in hydrostatic pressure
within Bowman's capsule or in plasma colloid osmotic pressure can alter
glomerular filtration rate. However, the major cause of changes in glomerular filtration rate is changes in glomerular-capillary hydrostatic
pressure.[1] How this pressure is regulated is described in a subsequent
section.

How is the rate of glomerular filtration measured (Fig. 7)? To
answer this question we use another substance (let us call it **W**) that is
freely filtered at the glomerulus but neither secreted nor reabsorbed by
the tubules:

$$\frac{\text{Mass of W excreted}}{\text{Time}} = \frac{\text{mass of W filtered}}{\text{time}} \tag{1}$$

Since the mass of any solute equals solute concentration times solvent
volume,

$$\frac{\text{Mass of W excreted}}{\text{Time}} = \frac{\text{urine conc of W} \times \text{urine volume}}{\text{time}} \tag{2}$$

Combining Eqs. (1) and (2):

$$U_W V = \frac{\text{mass of W filtered}}{\text{time}} \tag{3}$$

[1] See Deen et al., 1974 (Suggested Readings) for a different view.

where U_W = urine concentration and V = urine volume per time. Similarly, the mass of W filtered equals the product of the volume of plasma filtered into Bowman's capsule and the concentration of W per unit volume of filtrate. The volume of plasma filtered per unit time is, by definition, the *glomerular filtration rate* (GFR). Since W is freely filtered, the filtrate concentration of W is the same as the plasma concentration P_W. Therefore:

$$\frac{\text{Mass of W filtered}}{\text{time}} = P_W \times \text{GFR} \tag{4}$$

Combining Eqs. (3) and (4):

$$U_W V = P_W \times \text{GFR} \tag{5}$$

Three of the variables — V, P_W, and U_W — can be measured, and we can solve for GFR:

$$\text{GFR} = \frac{U_W V}{P_W} \tag{6}$$

The validity of the above analysis depends upon the following characteristics of W: Ex   Inulin

1 Freely filterable at the glomerulus
2 Not reabsorbed
3 Not secreted
4 Not synthesized by the tubules
5 Not broken down by the tubules

A polysaccharide called *inulin* (not insulin) completely fits this description and can be used for the determination of GFR. Consider the following hypothetical situation: In order to determine your patient's GFR, you infuse inulin at a rate sufficient to maintain his plasma concentration constant at 4 mg/liter. Urine collected over a 24-hr period has a volume of 2 liters and an inulin concentration of 360 mg/liter. What is the patient's GFR?

$$\text{GFR} = \frac{U_{In} V}{P_{In}}$$

$$\text{GFR} = \frac{360 \text{ mg/liter} \times 2 \text{ liters/24 hr}}{4 \text{ mg/liter}}$$

$$\text{GFR} = 180 \text{ liters/24 hr}$$

If any of the five criteria listed above were not valid for inulin, its use would not provide an accurate measure of GFR. For example, if inulin were secreted, which of the following statements would be true?

Calculated GFR would be higher than the true GFR.
Calculated GFR would be lower than the true GFR.

The first statement is correct because the mass of inulin excreted would represent both filtered *and* secreted inulin and therefore would be greater than the filtered inulin.

Once there is a means for measuring GFR, then it becomes possible to evaluate whether a substance is reabsorbed or secreted by the tubules. Thus, for any substance B which is freely filtered:

Mass of B filtered $= \text{GFR} \times P_B$
Mass of B excreted $= U_B V$
If $U_B V > \text{GFR} \times P_B$, then B must have been secreted
If $U_B V < \text{GFR} \times P_B$, then B must have been reabsorbed

Unfortunately, measuring GFR with inulin is inconvenient because inulin is not a normally occurring bodily substance and must therefore be administered intravenously at a continuous constant rate for several hours. Therefore, in clinical situations the indigenous substance *creatinine* is frequently used to *estimate* GFR. Creatinine is formed from muscle creatine and released into the blood at a fairly constant rate. Consequently, its blood concentration changes little during a 24-hr period so that one need obtain only a single blood sample and a 24-hr urine collection.

$$\text{Estimated GFR} = \frac{U_{Cr}V}{P_{Cr}}$$

This is only an estimated GFR because, in man, creatinine does not meet all five criteria; it is secreted by the tubules. It therefore overestimates the true GFR. However, the amount secreted is relatively small and the discrepancy is not very large. In a later section we will describe how measurement of plasma creatinine alone without any urine determinations can also be used to estimate GFR more crudely. Use of urea for the same purpose will also be described.

TUBULAR REABSORPTION

Many filterable plasma components are either completely absent from the urine or present in smaller quantities than were originally filtered at the glomerulus. This fact alone is sufficient to prove that these substances undergo tubular reabsorption. An idea of the magnitude and importance of these reabsorptive mechanisms can be gained from Table 3, which summarizes data for a few plasma components, all of which are

Table 3   Average Values for Components Handled by
Filtration and Reabsorption

Substance	Amount filtered per day	Amount excreted	% reabsorbed
Water, liters	180	1.8	99.0
Sodium, gm	630	3.2	99.5
Glucose, gm	180	0	100
Urea,* gm	56	28	50

* Urea handling is actually more complicated than just filtration and reabsorption. (See
Kokko, 1974, and Schmidt-Nielsen, 1970, in Suggested Readings for Chap. 5.)

handled by filtration and reabsorption. These are typical values for a
normal person on an average diet. There are at least three important
conclusions to be drawn from this table: (1) The quantities of material
entering the nephron via the glomerular filtrate are enormous, generally
larger than their total body stores. If reabsorption of water ceased but
filtration continued, the total plasma water would be urinated within 30
min. (2) The quantities of waste products, such as urea, which are
excreted in the urine are generally sizable fractions of the filtered
amounts. Thus, in mammals, coupling a large glomerular filtration rate
with a limited urea reabsorptive capacity permits rapid excretion of the
large quantities of this substance produced constantly as a result of protein breakdown. (3) In contrast to urea and other waste products, the
amount of most "useful" plasma components, e.g., water, electrolytes,
and glucose, which are excreted in the urine represent quite small fractions of the filtered amounts. For this reason one often hears the generalization that the kidney performs its regulatory function by *completely*
reabsorbing all of these biologically important materials and thereby
preventing their loss from the body. This is a misleading half-truth, the
refutation of which serves as an excellent opportunity for reviewing the
essential features of renal function and regulatory processes in general.
     Let us begin by pointing out the part of the generalization that is
true. Certain substances, notably glucose, are not normally excreted in
the urine because the amounts filtered are completely reabsorbed by the
tubules. But does such a system permit the kidneys to *regulate* the
plasma concentration of glucose, i.e., *set* it at some specific concentration? The following example will point out why the answer is no. Suppose the plasma glucose concentration is 100 mg/100 ml. Since reabsorption of this carbohydrate is complete, no glucose is lost from the
body via the urine, and the plasma concentration remains at 100 mg/100
ml. If, instead of 100 mg/100 ml, we set our hypothetical plasma glucose
concentration at 60 mg/100 ml, the analysis does not change; no glucose

is lost in the urine and the plasma glucose stays at 60 mg/100 ml. Obviously, the kidney is merely maintaining whatever plasma glucose concentration happens to exist and is not involved in the regulatory mechanisms by which the original setting of the plasma glucose was accomplished. It is not the kidney but primarily the liver and the endocrine system which set and regulate the plasma glucose concentration.[1] For comparison, consider what happens when a person drinks a lot of water: Within 1 to 2 hr all the excess has been excreted in the urine, chiefly, as we shall see, as the result of decreased renal tubular reabsorption of water. In this example the kidney is the effector organ of a reflex which maintains plasma water concentration within very narrow limits. The critical point is that for many plasma components, particularly the inorganic ions and water, the kidney does *not completely* reabsorb the total amounts filtered. The rates at which these substances are reabsorbed (and therefore the rates at which they are excreted) are constantly subject to physiological control. This ability to vary the reabsorption rates of water, sodium, calcium, phosphate, and many other substances and to vary the secretion rates of still others is really the essence of the kidney's ability to regulate the internal environment.

Types of Reabsorption

A bewildering variety of ions and molecules is found in the plasma. With the exception of the proteins (and a few ions or molecules bound to protein), these materials are all present in the glomerular filtrate, and most are reabsorbed to varying extents. It is essential to realize that tubular reabsorption is a qualitatively different process from glomerular filtration. The latter occurs by bulk flow, in which water and all dissolved free crystalloids move together. In contrast, there is little bulk flow across the tubular epithelium, mainly because the tubular epithelium is not porous enough to permit bulk flow.[2] Tubular reabsorption of various substances, then, is by more-or-less discrete tubular transport mechanisms, although in many cases a single reabsorptive system transports several different components, if they are similar in structure. For example, many of the simple carbohydrates are reabsorbed by the same system.

Transport processes can be categorized broadly as active or pas-

---

[1] Time and research give the lie to all generalizations. It is now known that the renal tubular cells actually *synthesize* glucose and release it into the blood during a prolonged fast. In this manner the kidneys do help set the plasma glucose concentration during prolonged fasting. This in no way detracts from the discussion above, which describes how glucose *reabsorption* does *not* contribute to the setting.

[2] Recently a considerable controversy has arisen concerning just how much proximal-tubular reabsorption might actually occur by bulk flow. (See Giebisch, 1974, in Suggested Readings for Chap. 5.)

sive, and there are examples of both in the kidney. The process is *passive* if no cellular energy is directly and specifically involved in the transport of the substance, i.e., if the substance moves downhill by simple or facilitated diffusion as a result of an electric or chemical concentration gradient. *Active* reabsorption, on the other hand, can produce net movement of the substance uphill against its concentration or electric gradient and therefore requires energy expenditure by the transporting cells.

Transport of any substance across the renal tubule involves a sequence of steps, for to cross the renal tubule, a substance must traverse not just one but a sequence of membranes. For example, to be reabsorbed, a sodium ion must gain entry to the tubular cell by crossing the cell membrane lining the lumen. It must then move through the cell's cytoplasm and cross the opposite cell membrane to enter the interstitial fluid. Finally, it must cross the basement membrane and capillary endothelium to enter the plasma. The entire process is known as *transepithelial transport* and occurs not only in the kidney but in the gastrointestinal tract and in other epithelial linings of the body.

In transepithelial transport the overall process is called *active* if one or more of the individual steps in the sequence is active. Sodium ions, for example, diffuse across the first tubular cell membrane (the luminal membrane) and through the cytoplasm of the cell (Fig. 10). They are then actively transported out of the cell and into the interstitial fluid, from which they gain entry into the capillary by the bulk flow process typical of all capillaries. (Note that this bulk flow into the peritubular capillaries does not contradict the previous statement that little or no bulk flow occurs from the tubular lumen across the epithelium and into the interstitial fluid.) Thus, three of the four steps are passive, but the crucial step is mediated by an active carrier process, and the overall process of sodium reabsorption is therefore said to be active.

Transport Maximum

Many of the active reabsorptive systems in the renal tubule can transport only limited amounts of material per unit time, primarily because the membrane carrier responsible for the transport becomes saturated. The classical example is the tubular transport process for glucose. As we know, normal persons do not excrete glucose in their urine because tubular reabsorption is complete. But it is possible to produce urinary excretion of glucose in a completely normal person merely by administering large quantities of glucose directly into one of his veins (Table 4).

Note that even after his plasma glucose concentration has doubled, his urine is still glucose-free, indicating that his *maximal tubular transport capacity T_m* for reabsorbing glucose has not yet been reached. But as the plasma glucose and the filtered load continue to rise, glucose finally appears in the urine. From this point on any further increase in

Table 4   Experimental Data Obtained for Calculation of Glucose T_m

Time, min	GFR, ml/min	P_G, mg/ml	Filtered glucose (GFR × P_G), mg/min	Excreted glucose ($U_G V$), mg/min	Reabsorbed glucose (filtered − excreted) mg/min
0	125	1.0	125	0	125
Begin glucose infusion					
26–40	125	2.0	250	0	250
100–110	125	4.0	500	125	375
130–140	125	5.0	625	250	375

Clearance

plasma glucose is accompanied by a proportionate increase in excreted glucose, because the T_m, which equals 375 mg/min, has now been reached. The tubules are now reabsorbing all the glucose they can, and any amount filtered in excess of this quantity cannot be reabsorbed and appears in the urine. This is precisely what occurs in the patient with diabetes mellitus. Because of a deficiency in pancreatic production of insulin, the patient's plasma glucose may rise to extremely high values. The filtered load of glucose becomes great enough to exceed the T_m, and glucose appears in the urine. There is nothing wrong with his tubular transport mechanism for glucose. It is simply unable to reabsorb the huge filtered load.

    To add one more level of complexity, let us return to the experiment in which glucose was infused. Additional data were obtained for minutes 60 to 100 but were not shown in Table 4. They are as follows:

Time, min	GFR, ml/min	P_G, mg/ml	Filtered glucose, mg/min	Excreted glucose, mg/min	Reabsorbed glucose, mg/min
60–80	125	2.8	350	20	330
80–100	125	3.5	436	76	360

Now we see that glucose began to appear in the urine *before* the true T_m of 375 mg/min was reached. There are several reasons for this *splay:* (1) An active transport mechanism shows kinetics analogous to those of enzyme systems so that maximal activity is substrate-dependent (in this case, glucose-dependent). (2) Not all nephrons have the same T_m for glucose. This last point is extremely important, for we too often fall into the habit of viewing the kidneys as one large nephron. The fact that there are really 2 million nephrons in the kidneys and that they are not completely identical in functional characteristics will be seen to have particularly important implications for renal sodium reabsorption.

Except for our experimental subject receiving intravenous glucose, the plasma glucose in normal persons never becomes high enough to cause urinary excretion of glucose because the reabsorptive capacity for glucose is much greater than necessary for normal filtered loads. However, for certain other substances, e.g., phosphate, the reabsorptive T_m is very close to the normal filtered load. The adaptive value inherent in such a relationship should be readily apparent from the following example: On a normal person the following data are obtained:

$$\text{Ingested } PO_4 = 20 \text{ mmol/day}$$
$$GFR = 180 \text{ liters/day}$$
$$\text{Plasma } PO_4 \text{ conc} = 1 \text{ mmol/liter}$$
$$\text{Filtered } PO_4 = 1 \times 180 = 180 \text{ mmol/day}$$
$$T_m \text{ for } PO_4 = 160 \text{ mmol/day}$$
$$\text{Excreted } PO_4 = 180 - 160 = 20 \text{ mmol/day}$$

Under these conditions the normal person remains in perfect phosphate balance since he is excreting precisely what he eats, and his plasma phosphate concentration therefore remains constant at 1 mmol/liter. If the next day he eats an unusually large quantity of phosphate and raises his plasma phosphate to 1.1 mmol/liter, the data are

$$GFR = 180 \text{ liters/day}$$
$$\text{Filtered } PO_4 = 1.1 \times 180 = 198 \text{ mmol/day}$$
$$T_m \text{ for } PO_4 = 160 \text{ mmol/day}$$
$$\text{Excreted } PO_4 = 198 - 160 = 38 \text{ mmol/day}$$

The very slight increase in plasma phosphate has resulted in a large increase in excreted phosphate and has eliminated the excess phosphate ingested. By this mechanism, depending on neither hormones nor nerves, the kidney can exert control over plasma phosphate concentration. We shall see that, in addition to this simplest of systems, more complex systems involving neural and hormonal components also exist for the regulation of phosphate and other electrolytes, but the basic relationship between filtered load and reabsorptive rate is the underlying principle for many of them.

The mechanisms for the transport of glucose and phosphate are similar in a number of ways: (1) They are both active transport systems; (2) they are both located in the proximal tubule; (3) they both manifest T_m's; and (4) they can be inhibited by other chemicals. The proximal tubule possesses similar active-T_m-limited-transport systems for a number of other important organic solutes, including amino acids, several Krebs cycle intermediates, lactate, acetoacetate and β-hydroxybutyrate, and others. In general, the T_m for each of the substances listed above, like that for glucose but unlike that for phosphate, is above the amount *normally* filtered. Accordingly, the kidneys normally protect against significant loss of the substance but do not help set its plasma concentration. However, just as was true for glucose in diabetic persons, under abnormal conditions the plasma concentration of any of these substances may become so increased as to cause the reabsorptive T_m for it to be exceeded and large quantities to be lost in the urine. Good examples are acetoacetate and β-hydroxybutyrate in patients with uncontrolled diabetes.

Protein

The proximal tubule also reabsorbs protein by an active process, perhaps involving pinocytosis. As mentioned above, there is a very small amount of protein in the glomerular filtrate. The exact normal concentration is unknown but is now thought to approximate 20 mg/liter, about 0.04 percent of plasma albumin concentration. Yet this is *not* negligible because of the huge volume of fluid filtered per day.

$$\begin{aligned}\text{Total filtered protein} &= \text{GFR} \times \text{filtrate conc of protein}\\ &= 180 \text{ liters/day} \times 20 \text{ mg/liter}\\ &= 3.6 \text{ gm/day}\end{aligned}$$

If none of this protein were reabsorbed, the entire 3.6 gm would be lost in the urine. In fact, virtually all of the filtered protein is reabsorbed so that the excretion of protein in the urine is normally only 100 mg/day. The mechanism by which protein is reabsorbed is easily saturated, so any large increase in filtered protein resulting from increased glomerular permeability can cause the excretion of large quantities of protein. For example, suppose that disease causes the glomeruli to allow 1 percent of the plasma albumin to be filtered:

$$\begin{aligned}\text{Filtered protein} &= \text{GFR} \times (50 \text{ gm/liter})(0.01)\\ &= 180 \text{ liters/day} \times 0.5 \text{ gm/liter}\\ &= 90 \text{ gm/day}\end{aligned}$$

This is far greater than the protein T_m, and large quantities of protein would be lost in the urine.

Urea

Just as glucose and phosphate provide excellent examples of actively transported solutes, urea provides an example of passive transport.

Since urea is freely filtered at the glomerulus, its concentration in the very first portion of the tubule is identical to its concentration in peritubular-capillary plasma. Then, as the fluid flows along the tubule, water reabsorption occurs, increasing the concentration of any intratubular solute not being reabsorbed at the same rate as the water. As a result, the concentration of urea in the tubular lumen becomes greater than the concentration of urea in the peritubular plasma. Accordingly, urea is able to diffuse passively down this concentration gradient from tubular lumen to peritubular capillary. Urea reabsorption is thus a passive process and completely dependent upon the reabsorption of water, which establishes the diffusion gradient. In man, urea reabsorption varies between 40 and 60 percent of the filtered urea, the lower figure holding when water reabsorption is low and the higher when it is high.[1]

Foreign Chemicals

Passive reabsorption is also of considerable importance for many foreign chemicals. The renal tubular epithelium acts in many respects as a lipid barrier; accordingly, highly lipid-soluble substances like urea can penetrate it fairly readily. Recall that one of the major determinants of lipid solubility is the polarity of a molecule; the more polar, the less lipid-soluble. Many drugs and environmental pollutants are nonpolar and, therefore, highly lipid-soluble. This makes their excretion from the body via the urine quite difficult, since they are filtered at the glomerulus and then, like urea, reabsorbed as water reabsorption causes their intratubular concentrations to increase. Fortunately, the liver transforms most of these substances to progressively more polar metabolites which, because of their reduced lipid solubility, are poorly reabsorbed by the tubules and can therefore be excreted. Polarity does not influence glomerular filtration.

TUBULAR SECRETION

Tubular secretory processes, which transport substances into the tubular lumen, i.e., in the direction opposite to tubular reabsorption, constitute a second pathway into the tubule, the first pathway being glomerular filtration. Like tubular reabsorptive processes, secretory transport may be either active or passive. Among the most important secretory processes are those for hydrogen ion, potassium, and ammonia. These will be discussed in detail later.

---

[1] Urea handling by the kidney is actually more complex than this simple filtration-reabsorption story suggests. (See Kokko, 1974, and Schmidt-Nielsen, 1970, in Suggested Readings for Chap. 5.)

There exist in the proximal tubule several secretory systems which are analogous to the proximal reabsorptive mechanisms described above in that they are active, T_m-limited, and can be inhibited by various agents. One transport mechanism secretes a variety of normally occurring and foreign organic acids, including paraaminohippuric acid and penicillin. A second system secretes many strong organic bases, both endogenous and foreign. There is at least one other distinct secretory pathway, and there may be more. The fact that these secretory mechanisms are relatively nondiscriminating and can transport foreign substances makes them important for the elimination from the body of drugs and other foreign environmental chemicals. Here again, the liver's metabolic transformations are frequently important. In the liver, many foreign (and endogenous) substances are conjugated with glucuronic acid or sulfate. These two categories of molecules are actively transported by the organic acid secretory pathway and are quite polar so that, following their secretion, they are not passively reabsorbed back into the blood.

URIC ACID: A COMPLEX EXAMPLE

To summarize and further illustrate some of the principles described above let us consider the renal handling of uric acid. Uric acid excretion in a normal man is found to be 700 mg/day; its concentration in plasma equals 5 mg/100 ml. How is uric acid handled by the kidney? First, we ascertain that uric acid is not protein-bound and that it is freely filterable. Therefore, we can now measure the quantity of uric acid filtered per unit time.

$$\text{Filtered uric acid} = \text{GFR} \times P_{\text{uric acid}}$$
$$= 180 \text{ liters/day} \times 50 \text{ mg/liter}$$
$$= 9,000 \text{ mg/day}$$

We can now say for certain that uric acid is reabsorbed by the tubules because the mass excreted per unit time is less than the mass filtered. Does this prove that uric acid is not secreted by the tubules? The answer is *no*. Secretion might be occurring at a much slower rate than reabsorption, which could therefore mask it. Indeed, such is the case with uric acid. If one administers certain drugs to block the secretory pathway, the excretion of uric acid decreases. Thus, we have a substance which is both reabsorbed and secreted. It is no wonder that the precise mechanisms and controls of uric acid excretion are still not clearly defined.

Study questions: 2 to 5

Chapter 3

Renal Clearance

OBJECTIVES

The student understands the principles and applications of clearance technique.

1 Defines the term clearance
2 Knows which clearances are used to measure GFR and ERPF
3 Lists the data required for clearance calculation
4 Given data, calculates C_{In}, C_{PAH}, C_{urea}, $C_{glucose}$, C_{Na}
5 Given data, calculates reabsorptive T_m for glucose and secretory T_m for PAH
6 Given data, calculates rates of reabsorption of Na, protein, glucose, phosphate, and other substances not secreted
7 Knows how to estimate GFR from C_{urea} and describes the limitations
8 Describes the limitation of C_{Cr} as a measure of GFR
9 Predicts whether a substance has undergone net reabsorption or net secretion from its clearance relative to that of inulin
10 Constructs the curve relating steady-state P_{Cr} to C_{Cr} or P_{urea} to C_{urea}; predicts the changes in P_{Cr} and P_{urea} given a known change in GFR; knows the limitations of this analysis, particularly with regard to urea

When we described how inulin could be used to measure GFR, we were actually describing a technique known as clearance. We should like to explain this concept more fully and to reemphasize its usefulness in evaluating renal function.

DEFINITION

First, let us define the term. The *clearance* of a substance is the *volume* of *plasma* from which that substance is *completely cleared* by the kidneys *per unit time*. Every substance in the blood has its own distinct clearance value, and the units are always in volume of plasma per time. Inulin offers an excellent first example. Since all excreted inulin must come from the plasma, one can see that a certain volume of plasma loses its inulin while flowing through the kidney; i.e., a certain volume of plasma is "cleared" of inulin. For inulin, this volume is obviously equal to the GFR, since none of the inulin contained in the glomerular filtrate returns to the blood (inulin is not reabsorbed) and since none of the plasma that escapes filtration loses any of its inulin (inulin is not secreted). Therefore, a volume of plasma equal to the GFR has been completely cleared of inulin. This volume is termed the inulin clearance and is expressed as C_{In}. Accordingly,

$$C_{In} = GFR$$

What is the glucose clearance? Glucose is freely filtered at the glomerulus so that all the glucose contained in the glomerular filtrate is lost *initially* from the plasma to the tubules. But, all of this filtered glucose is normally then reabsorbed; i.e., it is all returned to the plasma. The net result is that *no* plasma ends up losing glucose; the clearance of glucose is *zero*.

What is the phosphate clearance in the example cited earlier? The filtered PO_4 equals 180 mmol/day. Is this the phosphate clearance? The answer is *no*. Clearance does *not* designate a filtered mass. Indeed, it does not designate any mass; it is always a volume per time. The clearance of phosphate is defined as the volume of plasma completely cleared of phosphate per unit time. Is the clearance of phosphate, then, the GFR? Again the answer is *no*. Certainly, the filtered phosphate contained in the GFR is *temporarily* lost from the plasma but much of it is reabsorbed, in this example, 160 mmol/day, leaving only 20 mmol/day to be excreted in the urine. Is this the phosphate clearance?

Once again the answer is *no*. Clearance is not defined as mass excreted but rather as the volume of plasma supplying that mass per unit time. In other words, the phosphate clearance is the volume of plasma which supplies the excreted 20 mmol; it is this volume which is completely cleared of its phosphate. How much plasma has to be completely cleared of phosphate to supply the 20 mmol? We know from the data that the plasma phosphate concentration equals 1 mmol/liter. Therefore, it would take

$$\frac{20 \text{ mmol/day}}{1 \text{ mmol/liter}} = 20 \text{ liters/day}$$

to supply the excreted phosphate. Clearance of a substance really answers the question: How much plasma must be completely cleared to supply the excreted mass of that substance? This is really synonymous with the formal definition of clearance given above.

BASIC FORMULA

It should be evident, therefore, that the basic clearance formula is:

$$C_X = \frac{\text{mass of X excreted/time}}{P_X}$$
$$C_X = \frac{U_X V}{P_X}$$

C_{In} is a measure of GFR simply because the volume of plasma completely cleared of inulin, i.e., the volume from which the excreted inulin comes, is equal to the volume of plasma filtered. C_{PO_4} must be less than C_{In} because much of the filtered phosphate is reabsorbed; therefore, less plasma was cleared of phosphate than of inulin.

Thus, the following generalization emerges: Whenever the clearance of a freely filterable substance is less than the inulin clearance, tubular reabsorption of that substance must have occurred. This is simply another way of stating that whenever the mass of a substance excreted in the urine is less than the mass filtered during the same period of time, tubular reabsorption must have occurred. The phrase "freely filterable" is essential in the above generalization. Protein serves as an excellent example. The clearance of protein in a normal person is essentially zero, obviously lower than the C_{In}. However, this does not prove that protein is reabsorbed; the major reason for the zero clearance is that the protein is not filtered. Accordingly, in order to compare inulin clearance to the clearance of any completely or partially protein-bound substance (calcium, for example), one must use the free plasma concentration of the substance, rather than the total plasma concentration, in the clearance formula.

Is the clearance of creatinine in man higher or lower than that of inulin? The answer is higher. Like inulin, creatinine is freely filtered and not reabsorbed; therefore a volume of plasma equal to that of the GFR (i.e., the C_{In}) is completely cleared of creatinine. But, in addition, a small amount of creatinine is secreted. Therefore, some plasma in addition to that filtered is cleared of its creatinine by means of tubular secretion. The clearance formula is precisely the same as that for any other substance.

$$C_{Cr} = \frac{U_{Cr}V}{P_{Cr}}$$

Another generalization emerges: Whenever the clearance of a substance is greater than the inulin clearance, tubular secretion of that substance must have occurred. Again, this is merely another way of stating that whenever the excreted mass exceeds the filtered mass, secretion must be occurring.

Another substance secreted by the proximal tubules is the organic acid paraaminohippurate (PAH). PAH is also filtered at the glomerulus and, when its plasma concentration is fairly low, virtually all the PAH which escapes filtration is secreted. Since PAH is not reabsorbed, the net effect is that all the plasma supplying the nephrons is completely cleared of PAH. If PAH were completely cleared from all the plasma flowing through the *entire* kidney, then its clearance would measure the *total renal plasma flow*. However, about 10 to 15 percent of the total renal plasma flow supplies nonsecreting portions of the kidneys, such as peripelvic fat, and this plasma cannot, therefore, lose its PAH by secretion. Accordingly, the PAH clearance actually measures the so-called *effective renal plasma flow* (ERPF) and is approximately 85 to 90 percent of the true *total* renal plasma flow. The clearance formula for PAH is, of course:

$$C_{PAH} = \frac{U_{PAH}V}{P_{PAH}}$$

Once we have measured the ERPF, we can calculate easily the *effective renal blood flow* (ERBF):

$$ERBF = \frac{ERPF}{1 - V_c}$$

where V_c = the blood hematocrit, i.e., the fraction of blood occupied by erythrocytes.

It should be emphasized that C_{PAH} measures ERPF only when plasma PAH is fairly low. If plasma PAH were increased to a level so high that the PAH secretory T_m were exceeded, then PAH would not be completely removed from the plasma, and the use of its clearance as a measure of ERPF would be invalid. Another substance which is handled in a manner similar to PAH is diodrast; accordingly, C_D is also a measure of ERPF.

Urea clearance C_{urea} can be determined by the usual formula:

$$C_{urea} = \frac{U_{urea}V}{P_{urea}}$$

Is the urea clearance higher or lower than inulin clearance? The answer is lower. Urea, like inulin, is freely filterable, but approximately 50 percent of filtered urea is reabsorbed; therefore C_{urea} will be 50 percent of C_{In}. If the mass of urea reabsorbed were always exactly 50 percent of that filtered, could C_{urea} be used to estimate GFR? The answer is yes. One would merely multiply the C_{urea} by 2 to obtain a value equal to the GFR. Unfortunately, as described above, urea reabsorption varies between 40 and 60 percent of the filtered urea so that one cannot merely multiply by 2. Nonetheless, the clearance is easy to perform clinically and can be used as at least a crude indicator of glomerular function. The creatinine clearance is certainly a better way of evaluating GFR. But recall that, because of creatinine secretion, it is not completely accurate either.

PLASMA CREATININE AND UREA CONCENTRATION AS INDICATORS OF GFR CHANGES

As described previously, the creatinine clearance is a close approximation of the GFR and is therefore a valuable clinical determination.

$$C_{Cr} = \frac{U_{Cr}V}{P_{Cr}}$$

In practice, however, it is far more common to measure plasma creatinine alone and to use this as an indicator of GFR. This approach is justified by the fact that most excreted creatinine gains entry to the tubule by filtration. If we ignore the small amount secreted, there should be an excellent inverse correlation between plasma creatinine and GFR, as shown by the following example: A normal person's plasma creatinine is 10 mg/liter. It remains stable because each day he excretes the same amount of creatinine he produces. One day his GFR suddenly decreases permanently by 50 percent because of a blood clot in the renal artery. On that day he filters only 50 percent as much creatinine as normal so

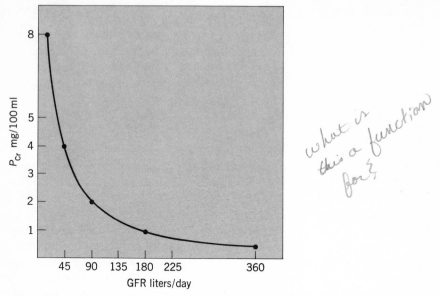

Figure 8   Steady state relationship between GFR and plasma creatinine (assuming no creatinine is secreted).

that creatinine excretion is also reduced by 50 percent. (We are ignoring the small contribution of secreted creatinine.) Therefore, assuming no change in creatinine production, he goes into positive creatinine balance, and his plasma creatinine rises. But despite the persistent 50 percent GFR reduction, his plasma creatinine does not indefinitely continue to rise; rather, it stabilizes at 20 mg/liter, i.e., after it has doubled. At this point he once again is able to excrete creatinine at the normal rate and so remains stable. The reason is that the 50 percent GFR reduction has been counterbalanced by the increase in plasma creatinine, and filtered creatinine is again normal.

Original normal state: Filtered creatinine = 10 mg/liter × 180 liters/day
$$= 1,800 \text{ mg/day}$$
New steady state: Filtered creatinine = 20 mg/liter × 90 liters/day
$$= 1,800 \text{ mg/day}$$

What if the GFR then fell to 30 liters/day? Again creatinine retention would occur until a new steady state had been established, i.e., until he is again filtering 1,800 mg/day. What would the new plasma creatinine be?

$$1,800 \text{ mg/day} = P_{Cr} \times 30 \text{ liters/day}$$
$$P_{Cr} = 60 \text{ mg/liter}$$

It should now be clear why a single plasma creatinine is a reasonable indicator of GFR (Fig. 8). Of course, it is not completely accurate for three reasons: (1) Some creatinine is secreted. (2) There is no way of knowing exactly what his original creatinine was when GFR was normal. (3) Creatinine production may not remain completely unchanged.

Since urea is also handled by filtration, the same type of analysis would indicate that measurement of plasma urea concentration could serve as an indicator of GFR. However, it is much less accurate because the range of normal plasma urea concentration varies widely, depending upon protein intake and changes in tissue catabolism, and because urea is reabsorbed to a *variable* degree. The fact that it is reabsorbed would not interfere with its use as an indicator if the reabsorption were always a *fixed* percent of the filtered mass.

Study questions: **6** to **12**

Chapter 4

Renal Hemodynamics

OBJECTIVES

The student understands the control of renal hemodynamics.
1 States the formula relating flow, pressure, and resistance
2 Knows the normal rates of the GFR and RBF and defines filtration fraction
3 Defines autoregulation of RBF and GFR; states the condition in which "pure" autoregulation can be observed
4 Describes the role of the sympathetic nervous system
5 Describes how changes in filtration fraction occur
6 Defines distribution of flow (cortex-medulla and cortex-cortex)
7 .Predicts the direction of change of GFR under a variety of situations such as hypotension, reduced plasma protein, and ureteral occlusion

The total blood flow to the kidneys is approximately 1.1 liters/min. Thus, the kidneys receive 20 to 25 percent of the total cardiac output (5 liters/min) even though their combined weight is less than 1 percent of the total body weight! Given a normal hematocrit of 0.45, the total renal plasma flow = 0.55 × 1.1 liters/min = 605 ml/min. You now should be able to calculate what fraction of the plasma entering the kidneys is filtered into Bowman's capsule. The answer is 20 percent. Recall that the GFR equals 125 ml/min. Therefore, of the 605 ml of plasma that enters the glomeruli via the afferent arterioles, 125/605, or 20 percent, filters into Bowman's capsule, the remaining 480 ml passing via the efferent arterioles into the peritubular capillaries. This ratio is known as the *filtration fraction*.

Recall that the basic equation for blood flow through any organ is

$$\text{Organ blood flow} = \frac{\Delta P}{R}$$

where ΔP = mean arterial pressure minus venous pressure for that organ
R = resistance to flow through that organ
Recall also that, normally, the major determinant of resistance is the radii of the arterioles within that organ. It should be evident, therefore, that renal blood flow is determined mainly by the mean arterial pressure and the renal arteriolar tonus.

MEAN ARTERIAL PRESSURE AND AUTOREGULATION

The renal circulation manifests quite markedly the phenomenon of autoregulation. The rate of blood flow through the kidney is relatively constant in the face of changes in mean arterial pressure — at least in the face of mean-arterial-pressure changes that range between 80 and 180 mmHg. Look again at the basic cardiovascular equation above. This equation predicts that, if the pressure gradient is increased by 50 percent and resistance stays constant, blood flow will increase 50 percent. In the kidney, however, such is not the case. If one isolates a kidney experimentally and perfuses it with blood by means of a pump, one can demonstrate that a 50-percent increase in pressure gradient produces less than a 10-percent increase in blood flow. There is only one possible explanation: Resistance in the kidney does *not* stay constant as *arterial* pressure increases. Rather, resistance automatically increases. The renal arterioles constrict when the arterial pressure increases; therefore, blood flow remains relatively unchanged. The intrarenal mechanism mediating these arteriolar changes has been the subject of considerable investigation and controversy, but no completely satisfactory explanation has been found.

This entire discussion applies not only to RBF but to GFR, which also shows only small changes in the face of large changes in arterial pressure. There are several reasons for the fact that GFR, as well as RBF, is autoregulated. One of the most important is that the *afferent* arterioles are the major site of autoregulatory resistance changes in the face of arterial-pressure changes; accordingly, glomerular-capillary pressure (and, therefore, net filtration pressure) remains relatively unchanged.[1] For example, a rise in arterial pressure triggers enhanced afferent-arteriolar constriction, thereby increasing the pressure drop between the arteries and glomerular capillaries and preventing the transmission of the increased arterial pressure to the glomerulus.

What is the adaptive value of autoregulation? As in any other organ, it helps ameliorate blood-flow changes in the face of arterial-pressure fluctuations, but it also serves a unique role in the kidney, namely the blunting of the large changes in solute and water excretion which could otherwise occur (because of large GFR changes) whenever arterial pressure changed. This is the adaptive value of GFR autoregulation. Recall that the normal net filtration pressure in the glomeruli is only about 5 to 6 mmHg. Accordingly, even relatively minor changes in arterial pressure could cause marked increases or decreases in glomerular-capillary pressure and GFR were not these changes effectively blunted by automatically elicited changes in afferent-arteriolar tonus.

Having pointed out the value of autoregulation, we must now emphasize three facts: (1) Autoregulation is not perfect. RBF and GFR *do change* when renal arterial pressure is changed, but they change to a much smaller degree than they would if autoregulation did not exist. (2) Autoregulation is virtually absent at mean arterial pressures below 70 mmHg and therefore cannot blunt GFR and RBF changes below this point. (3) Despite autoregulation, RBF and GFR *can be altered considerably,* even when the arterial pressure is within the autoregulatory range, by the factors to be described next.

SYMPATHETIC NERVOUS SYSTEM

In the above discussion of autoregulation, we set up artificial experimental conditions in which renal blood pressure could be changed without altering blood pressure in the other arteries of the body. In order to demonstrate autoregulation clearly, this was necessary because, when the systemic arterial pressure decreases in the *intact* organism, a second variable is brought into play. This variable is the reflexly mediated increased sympathetic outflow to the kidneys (as well as increased circulating levels of epinephrine). This sympathetic input causes renal

---

[1] A second reason is described by Deen et al., 1974. (See Suggested Readings, Chap. 4.)

arteriolar constriction and decreases both RBF and GFR. Thus, although autoregulation blunts the *direct* effects on the kidney of changes in perfusion pressure, *sympathetic reflexes* can cause changes in renal hemodynamics when systemic arterial pressure is altered. As we shall see, such responses are importantly involved in the renal regulation of sodium and water excretion. If sympathetic input were solely to the afferent arteriole, then the decreases in GFR and RBF induced by increased sympathetic tone would be approximately the same. However, both afferent and efferent arterioles are constricted when sympathetic tone is increased; therefore, GFR tends not to decrease as much as

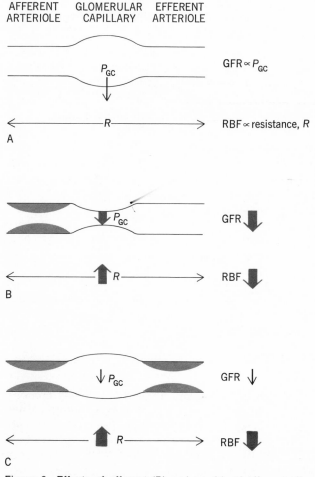

AFFERENT   GLOMERULAR   EFFERENT
ARTERIOLE   CAPILLARY   ARTERIOLE

Figure 9   Effects of afferent (B) and combined afferent-efferent (C) arteriolar constriction on GFR and RBF. Adding efferent constriction lowers RBF still further (because total resistance is increased) but restores GFR toward normal. Filtration fraction is, therefore, increased.

RBF. The reason for this is that, because the efferent arterioles lie beyond the glomerulus, an increase in their resistance tends to raise glomerular-capillary pressure—just the opposite of the effect of afferent-arteriolar constriction (see Fig. 9). In other words, increased sympathetic tone to the kidneys usually increases the filtration fraction GFR/RPF by causing relatively greater reductions in RPF than in GFR.

INTRARENAL DISTRIBUTION OF BLOOD FLOW

Total renal blood flow can be measured readily either by clearance techniques or by more direct methods such as flow probes. However, measurement of *regional* blood flows within the kidney has proven to be quite difficult. One well-established fact is that the cortex receives more than 90 percent of the total renal blood flow, the medulla receiving only a very small amount of blood. (The adaptive value of this for urine concentration will be discussed later.) The paucity of medullary blood flow is due to the resistance offered by the vasa recta, but it is not yet possible to quantitate the contributions of the multiple factors (vessel length, blood viscosity, neural tone, chemical mediators, etc.) which cause the resistance in the vasa recta to be higher than in the other intrarenal vessels.

Even more difficult to analyze is the relative distribution of blood flow within the cortex between the juxtamedullary nephrons and the superficial nephrons. It does seem clear that differences exist and are subject to physiological control. The possible significance of this phenomenon for the renal handling of sodium and water is discussed below. The factors which control this distribution have not been clearly determined, although differential sympathetic outflow to the arterioles of the superficial and juxtamedullary areas of the cortex seems to be at least one important mechanism.

HUMORAL CONTROL OF RENAL VASCULATURE

The renal vasculature is sensitive to many normally occurring humoral substances, such as epinephrine, angiotensin, antidiuretic hormone, histamine, bradykinin, and prostaglandins. But whether any of these substances actually participates in the physiological control of renal blood flow is unclear.

Study questions: **13** to **14**

Chapter 5

Basic Renal Processes for Sodium, Chloride, and Water

OBJECTIVES

The student understands the basic renal processes for sodium, chloride, and water.

1 Calculates or lists the quantities of sodium, chloride, and water normally filtered, reabsorbed, and excreted per day

2 Describes the nature (active or passive) of the process for each substance and the interrelationships between them, i.e., the forces involved; defines transtubular PD

3 Describes the pathway followed by the transported fluid; defines tight junctions and intercellular spaces

4 Lists the percentages of sodium and water reabsorbed by each nephron segment

5 Knows the fluid osmolarity in each nephron segment during water diuresis and antidiuresis

6 Describes the mechanism of action of osmotic diuretics

7 Describes the countercurrent multiplier system for urine concentration; states the transport and permeability characteristics of the ascending and descending limbs and the collecting ducts

8 States the net loss or gain of solute and water for the two limbs of the loop and the collecting duct; states the action of ADH and the nephron sites on which it acts

9 Describes the medullary circulation and its functioning as a counter-current exchanger

10 Describes the obligatory relationships between sodium and water excretion

Table 1 was a typical balance sheet for water; Table 5 is the same for sodium. The excretion of sodium via the skin and gastrointestinal tract is normally quite small but may increase markedly during severe sweating, burns, vomiting, diarrhea, or hemorrhage. Control of the renal excretion of sodium and water constitutes the most important mechanism for the regulation of body sodium and water. The excretory rates of these substances can be varied over an extremely wide range. For example, a consumer of gross amounts of salt may ingest 20 to 25 gm of sodium chloride per day; whereas a patient on a low-salt diet may ingest only 50 mg. The normal kidney can readily alter its excretion of salt over this range. Similarly, urinary water excretion can be varied physiologically from approximately 400 ml/day to 25 liters/day depending upon whether one is lost in the desert or participating in a beer-drinking contest.

Sodium, chloride, and water are all freely filterable at the glomerulus and undergo considerable tubular reabsorption — normally, more than 99 percent (see Table 3) — but no tubular secretion. Indeed, the vast majority of all renal energy utilization goes to accomplish this enormous reabsorptive task. The tubular mechanisms for reabsorption of these substances can be summarized by three generalizations which apply to all nephron segments with the probable exception of the ascending loop of Henle (see below): (1) The reabsorption of sodium is an active process; i.e., it is carrier-mediated, requires an energy supply, and can occur against an electrochemical gradient. (2) The reabsorption of chlo-

Table 5 Normal Routes of
Sodium Chloride Intake
and Loss

Route	gm/day
Intake	
Food	10.5
Output	
Sweat	0.25
Feces	0.25
Urine	10.0
Total output	10.5

ride is primarily by passive diffusion and depends upon the active reabsorption of sodium. (3) The reabsorption of water also is passive and
depends upon the active reabsorption of sodium. Thus, active tubular
sodium reabsorption is the primary force which results in reabsorption
of chloride and water as well. As mentioned above, it is likely that the
ascending loop of Henle constitutes an exception to the generalizations.
Present evidence suggests that, in this nephron segment, the first two
generalizations are reversed; i.e., chloride reabsorption is the primary,
active process, and sodium reabsorption is by passive diffusion, dependent upon the active chloride movement. Generalization three still holds
in that water reabsorption is passive and dependent upon active ion
transport (except that, in this case, the actively transported ion is chloride rather than sodium). In describing below the mechanisms by which
ion-ion and ion-water movements are coupled, we shall do so in terms of
active sodium transport, since this process is the key event in most
nephron segments.

SODIUM-WATER COUPLING

As a first approach to understanding the sodium-water coupling mechanisms, let us treat the tubular-epithelium–peritubular-capillary barrier in
a highly simplified manner, as a single membrane separating the tubular-
lumen fluid from the peritubular-capillary plasma. This membrane
possesses an active sodium pump which transports sodium across the
membrane, i.e., actively reabsorbs sodium ions. How is the passive reabsorption of water coupled to the active transport of sodium? Since the concentrations of all crystalloids are identical in plasma and in Bowman's
capsular fluid, in the very first portion of the proximal tubule no significant transtubular concentration differences exist for sodium, chloride, or
water. (Transtubular, here, means between tubular-lumen fluid and peritubular-capillary plasma.) As the fluid flows down the tubule, sodium is
actively transported across the tubular epithelium. What does this do to
the water concentration of the tubular fluid? Obviously, this removal of
solute from the tubular fluid raises its water concentration, i.e., lowers
its osmolarity below that of plasma. Thus a transtubular water concentration gradient is created which constitutes a driving force for water
reabsorption via osmosis. If the water permeability of the tubular epithelium is very high, water molecules are reabsorbed passively, almost as
rapidly as the actively transported sodium ions, so that the tubular fluid
is only slightly more dilute than plasma. Theoretically, in this manner almost all the filtered sodium and water could be reabsorbed, and the final
urine would still have approximately the same osmolarity as plasma.
However, this reabsorption of water can occur only if the tubular epithelium is highly permeable to water. No matter how great the water con-

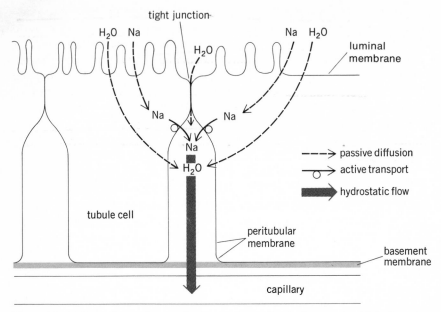

Figure 10   Pathway for sodium and water reabsorption in the proximal tubule.

centration gradient, water cannot move if the epithelium is impermeable to it. In reality, the permeability of the more distal portions of the nephron is subjected to physiological controls that we shall describe in detail below.

Although the above description is correct in its essentials, it is over-simplified because it ignores the anatomical pathways followed by sodium and water during reabsorption. These have recently been the subject of considerable investigation. As we shall see, they have important implications for the control of these processes. At present, the following schema seems most likely, at least for the proximal tubule (Fig. 10). Adjacent cells of the proximal tubule are connected at their luminal borders by *tight junctions,* which are very short. Behind these tight junctions are intercellular spaces filled with interstitial fluid. Sodium diffuses into the cells from the lumen and is actively pumped into these intercellular spaces, thereby generating a zone of local hyperosmolarity which osmotically attracts water across the cell membranes or tight junctions. As fluid accumulates in the intercellular spaces, the hydrostatic pressure increases and forces the fluid along the intercellular spaces. Finally, the fluid is moved from the intercellular spaces, across the basement membrane, and into the peritubular capillaries by the net balance of hydrostatic and colloid osmotic pressure forces acting across the capillaries.

This model explains a heretofore puzzling problem concerning transepithelial transport in the proximal tubule, as well as in the gut, gallbladder, and other epithelia. Measurements of proximal-luminal fluid have consistently revealed only negligible osmolarity differences between this fluid and peritubular plasma. Yet, the entire concept of water passively following sodium demands an osmotic gradient to drive water movement. Now we can see that the critical osmotic gradient is between the lumen and the intercellular space, the latter being hyperosmotic.

SODIUM-CHLORIDE COUPLING

How is the passive reabsorption of chloride coupled to the active transport of sodium? There are at least two mechanisms responsible for this coupling. The first mechanism is precisely the same as that previously described for urea. As water moves out of the tubule (secondary to sodium transport), all solutes in the tubule not subject to active transport will increase in concentration. By this means, a chloride transtubular concentration gradient is established, which acts as a driving force for chloride reabsorption by passive diffusion. (You should now recognize that the reabsorption of urea, just as that of chloride, is indirectly coupled to sodium transport via the latter's effect on water reabsorption.)

The second mechanism coupling passive chloride reabsorption to active sodium transport is the *electric potential difference* (PD) which exists across the tubular epithelium. In all nephron segments, with the exception of the loop of Henle, the tubular-lumen side of the epithelium is negatively charged compared to the peritubular side. The magnitude of this PD varies throughout the tubule, ranging from 0 to -4 mV in the proximal tubule to -40 to -60 mV in the distal tubule. One major contributing factor to this potential is undoubtedly the active reabsorption of sodium. Just on an intuitive level, it should be evident that the active transport of positively charged sodium ions out of the lumen tends to leave the inside of the lumen negatively charged as long as anion transport lags even slightly behind. A systematic analysis of the precise origins of this transtubular PD is beyond the scope of this presentation. What is more important for present purposes is the fact that this PD exists, is contributed to by active sodium transport, and constitutes a driving force for passive chloride reabsorption.

We have, then, both an electric and a chemical (i.e., concentration) difference favoring passive chloride reabsorption. In the proximal tubule, where the PD is very small, the concentration difference created by sodium-coupled water transport is most important. In the distal tubules and collecting ducts a very large PD exists and constitutes the major driving force for chloride movement. In both cases, however, the chloride movement is passive and is ultimately dependent upon active sodium reabsorption. (It should be possible for the reader to guess what the situation is in the ascending loop of Henle. In the ascending loop, chloride transport is the *active* primary event and causes the lumen to be *positively* charged relative to the peritubular fluid, and this constitutes a driving force for the passive reabsorption of sodium.)

With these generalizations as guides, let us now discuss some of the distinct characteristics of the individual nephron segments relative to salt and water handling.

PROXIMAL TUBULE

The proximal tubule is the site of greatest sodium and water reabsorption. Approximately 65 percent of the total filtered sodium and water is reabsorbed by the time the fluid has reached the end of the proximal tubule. Its water permeability is always very great, so passive water reabsorption keeps pace with active sodium reabsorption. What, therefore, is the concentration of sodium at the end of the proximal tubule? The answer is: almost equal to the plasma sodium concentration. It is true that 65 percent of the mass of sodium filtered has been reabsorbed but so has almost 65 percent of the filtered water. Therefore, the *concentration* of *sodium*, as opposed to the *mass,* remains virtually unchanged during fluid passage through the proximal tubule.

What is the *osmolarity* of the fluid at the end of the proximal tubule? Virtually the same as plasma (300 mOsm/liter), the logic being the same as for the question above concerning sodium concentration. Sodium and its associated anions, chloride and bicarbonate, constitute 90 to 95 percent of the osmotically active solute of plasma. (We shall see later that bicarbonate reabsorption in the proximal tubule also keeps pace with sodium.) Therefore, their concentrations normally determine the osmolarity of the proximal tubular fluid.

To summarize, during passage through the proximal tubule, approximately 65 percent of the sodium, chloride, and water are reabsorbed, but the sodium concentration and osmolarity of the fluid remain essentially the same as in plasma. This fact raises an interesting question: If sodium concentration is approximately plasmalike throughout the proximal tubule, how do we know that sodium reabsorption is an active process? To prove active transport, we must demonstrate net transport against an electrochemical gradient; yet the proximal tubule has only a small transtubular electric gradient, and we normally find no concentration gradient. Assuming that sodium transport really is active, then the reason that no concentration gradient is normally created is that water reabsorption keeps up with sodium. We must create an experimental situation in which water movement is retarded; in such a case, sodium reabsorption will get well ahead of water reabsorption, intraluminal sodium concentration will fall, and active sodium transport will have been demonstrated. This condition occurs in the presence of an osmotic diuretic.

An *osmotic diuretic* is a substance which retards water (and sodium) reabsorption merely because of its osmotic contribution to the tubular fluid. Recall that sodium and its anions normally constitute most of the osmotically active solute in plasma. Let us alter the situation by administering to a dog large amounts of the sugar mannitol so that its plasma concentration equals 100 mOsm/liter. Mannitol is freely filtered at the glomerulus but is not reabsorbed. In the first portion of the proximal tubule, therefore, mannitol will contribute 100 mOsm/liter. As sodium is actively reabsorbed, the total osmolarity of the proximal-tubular fluid begins to decrease and water therefore passively follows the sodium. However, because the mannitol cannot be reabsorbed, its concentration increases as water is reabsorbed. This type of concentrating effect has been previously described for chloride and for urea and obviously will apply to any solute whose reabsorption is slower than that of water. The crucial difference between our experimental conditions and the normal state is that the normally present "lagging" solutes either are present in very small concentration, or like chloride, follow closely behind the water. The mannitol, in contrast, is present in a very large concentration and is not reabsorbed at all. Accordingly, as its concentration raises as a result of water reabsorption, its osmotic presence retards the further reabsorption of water. Thus, passive water movement is prevented from keeping up with active sodium transport. The result is that sodium concentration in the lumen decreases below plasma sodium concentration, and proof of net transport against a concentration gradient is obtained.

We would not have burdened the reader with this analysis if our sole purpose were to show how the active nature of proximal sodium transport was proven. Far more important for clinical medicine is the fact that osmotic diuresis occurs in several disease states, including diabetes mellitus. Glucose is normally completely reabsorbed in the proximal tubule. But in the patient with uncontrolled diabetes mellitus, the filtered load may exceed the glucose T_m, and large quantities of glucose may remain unreabsorbed in the proximal tubule. Just like mannitol in the above example, the presence of this glucose retards water reabsorption and causes an osmotic diuresis. In such a patient, the filtered load of the ketone bodies, acetoacetate and β-hydroxybutyrate, may also exceed the T_m's for these substances so that they also contribute to the osmotic diuresis.

In our discussion of osmotic diuresis we have emphasized the poor reabsorption and increased excretion of water which occurs. Less easy to understand is the fact that osmotic diuretics cause the excretion of large quantities of sodium (and chloride) as well as of water. The major reason for this phenomenon illustrates another important characteristic of renal sodium transport: Simultaneously with the *active* transport of sodium out of the tubule, there are occurring quite large *passive* fluxes of sodium in both directions, since the tubule is quite permeable to sodium. But is there a *net passive flux* into or out of the proximal tubule? Normally there is very little, since there is no significant transtubular concentration difference for sodium and since the electric potential difference across the proximal tubule is quite small. Therefore, the opposing *passive* fluxes of sodium simply cancel each other out, leaving only the outwardly directed *active*-sodium-transport pathway to account for overall *net* sodium movement. However, in the presence of an osmotic diuretic, this situation is altered; because the osmotic diuretic retards water reabsorption, active sodium reabsorption causes the intratubular sodium concentration to decrease as described above. As a result there is a sodium concentration gradient favoring *net passive* sodium movement from peritubular plasma to lumen. This net passive influx opposes the active outflux, and so the *overall net* removal of sodium from the proximal-tubular lumen is diminished. This is one of the reasons that osmotic diuretics such as mannitol (or glucose in the diabetic) induce the excretion of large quantities of sodium (and chloride) as well as water. The impression should not be given that osmotic diuretics inhibit water and electrolyte reabsorption in the proximal tubule only. In fact, a similar type of inhibition occurs along the entire nephron and is quantitatively most important in the loop of Henle.

LOOP OF HENLE

The loops of Henle normally reabsorb approximately 25 percent of the filtered sodium and chloride and 15 percent of the filtered water. What percentages of the filtered sodium and water therefore enter the distal tubule? The answer is: 10 and 20 percent, respectively, since one must add the quantities reabsorbed by the loop to those already reabsorbed by the proximal tubule to obtain the total quantities unreabsorbed prior to the distal tubule.

    As mentioned earlier, the reabsorption of sodium, chloride, and water in the ascending loop is unusual in that chloride is the active process which secondarily induces passive reabsorption of sodium. However, the specific interactions between sodium, chloride, and water are considerably more complex than in the proximal tubule, and we shall return to them in a subsequent section. For the moment, it is sufficient to emphasize that the loop, unlike the proximal tubule, reabsorbs considerably more solute than water.

DISTAL TUBULE AND COLLECTING DUCT

Sodium, chloride, and water reabsorption continue along these last tubular segments so that the final urine normally contains less than 1 percent of the total filtered sodium. What is the osmolarity and sodium concentration of the fluid entering the distal tubule from the loop? Because more solute than water was reabsorbed in the loop, both the osmolarity and sodium concentration of the early distal fluid are well below those of plasma. The way in which osmolarity changes as the fluid flows along the distal tubule depends mainly upon the water permeability of the tubule. If the water permeability is very great, the fluid equilibrates with the plasma in the peritubular capillaries surrounding the distal tubules and becomes isoosmotic (300 mOsm/liter). Thus, after equilibrium has occurred, the late distal tubule behaves similarly to the proximal, reabsorbing equivalent amounts of solute and water. In contrast, when water permeability is low, the hypoosmotic fluid entering the distal tubule may become even more hypoosmotic as it flows along the tubule, and sodium reabsorption continues unaccompanied by equivalent water reabsorption. Under these conditions, sodium concentrations of the tubular fluid may fall to barely detectable levels.

The water permeability of the collecting ducts shows the same variability as that of the distal tubule. Thus, in the presence of low permeability, the highly dilute fluid delivered from the distal tubules remains dilute as it flows through the collecting ducts. In contrast, when the water permeability of the distal tubule and collecting duct is very great, the isoosmotic fluid leaving the distal tubule is progressively concentrated in its passage through the collecting ducts. This should come as a surprise since, on the basis of what has been so far described, one ought to conclude that the fluid would merely remain isoosmotic. The explanation will be given in the next section.

The major determinant of distal and collecting-duct water permeability is the hormone known as vasopressin, or antidiuretic hormone (ADH). The second name is preferable because it describes the effect of the hormone's action—antidiuresis (i.e., against a high urine volume). In the absence of ADH the tubular water permeability is very low, but sodium reabsorption may proceed normally because ADH has no significant effect on sodium reabsorption. Thus water is unable to follow and remains in the tubule to be excreted as a large volume of urine. On the other hand, in the presence of maximum amounts of ADH, the tubular water permeability of these last nephron segments is very great, and the final urine volume is small—less than 1 percent of the total filtered water. Of course, the tubular response to ADH is not all-or-none, like an action potential, but shows graded increases as the plasma concentration of ADH is increased over a certain range, thus permitting fine adjustments of water permeability and excretion. ADH exerts its action by inducing increased activity of cyclic AMP in the tubular cells, but the mechanism by which cyclic AMP increases tubular water permeability is still not clear.

It should now be easy to understand how the kidneys produce a final urine having the same osmolarity as that of plasma or one having a lower osmolarity than plasma (hypoosmotic urine), the latter occurring whenever water reabsorption lags behind solute reabsorption, i.e., when plasma ADH is reduced. Clearly the formation of a hypoosmotic urine is a good compensation for an excess of water in the body.

But how can the kidneys ever produce a hyperosmotic urine, i.e., a urine having an osmolarity greater than that of plasma? For this to occur does not water reabsorption have to get ahead of solute reabsorption? How can this happen if water reabsorption is always secondary to solute, particularly salt reabsorption? It would seem that if our three generalizations are not to be violated, then the kidneys cannot produce a hyperosmotic urine. Yet, as we have mentioned, they do. Indeed the final urine may be as concentrated as 1,400 mOsm/liter compared with a plasma osmolarity of 300 mOsm/liter. Moreover, this concentrated urine is produced without violating the three generalizations.

URINE CONCENTRATION: THE MEDULLARY COUNTERCURRENT SYSTEM

The ability of the kidneys to produce concentrated urine is not merely an academic problem. It is a major determinant of one's ability to survive without water. The human kidney can produce a maximal urinary concentration of 1,400 mOsm/liter. The urea, sulfate, phosphate, and other waste products (plus the small number of nonwaste ions) which must be excreted each day amount to approximately 600 mOsm. Therefore, the water required for their excretion constitutes an obligatory water loss and equals:

$$\frac{600 \text{ mOsm/day}}{1,400 \text{ mOsm/liter}} = 0.444 \text{ liter/day} \qquad \text{Obligatory } H_2O \text{ loss}$$

As long as the kidneys are functioning, excretion of this volume of urine will occur, despite the absence of water intake. In a sense, a person lacking access to water may literally urinate himself to death due to fluid depletion. If we could produce a urine with an osmolarity of 6,000 mOsm/liter, then only 100 ml of water need be lost obligatorily each day, and survival time would be greatly expanded. A desert rodent, the kangaroo rat, does just that. This animal never even drinks water because the water produced by oxidation is ample for his needs.

Countercurrent Multiplication

The kidneys produce concentrated urine by a complex interaction of events involving the so-called *countercurrent multiplier system* residing in the loop of Henle. Recall that the loop of Henle, which is interposed between the proximal and distal convoluted tubules, is a hair pin loop extending into the renal medulla. Let us list the critical characteristics of this loop.

1 The ascending limb of the loop of Henle[1] (i.e., the limb leading to the distal tubule) *actively* transports chloride out of the tubular lumen into the surrounding interstitium. It is also quite permeable to sodium. Therefore, the active chloride transport causes the passive movement of sodium out of the lumen, and we shall refer to the overall process as sodium chloride transport. However, the ascending limb is *relatively* impermeable to both chloride and water, so that *passive* fluxes of these substances into or out of it are small.

2 The descending limb of the loop of Henle (i.e., the limb into which drains fluid from the proximal tubule) does *not actively* transport either chloride or sodium. It is the only tubular segment that does not. Moreover, it has a very great permeability to water but is relatively impermeable to the ions.

Keeping these characteristics in mind, imagine the loop of Henle filled with a stationary column of fluid supplied by the proximal tubule. At first, the concentration everywhere would be 300 mOsm/liter, since fluid leaving the proximal tubule is isoosmotic to plasma.

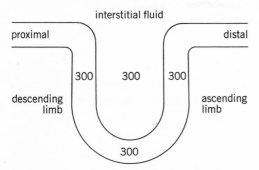

Now let the active pump in the ascending limb transport sodium chloride into the interstitium until a limiting gradient (say 200 mOsm/liter) is established between ascending-limb fluid and interstitium.

[1] The ascending loop of Henle is not a structurally homogenous segment. It is very thin (as is the descending loop) from the bend in the loop up to the outer medulla, where it becomes much thicker. This structural difference almost certainly reflects functional differences as well. However, for simplicity, we present the physiological characteristics of the thicker portion only. (See Kokko, 1974, in Suggested Readings for Chap. 5.)

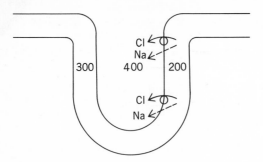

A limiting gradient is reached because the ascending limb is not *completely* impermeable to chloride. Accordingly, passive back flux into the lumen counterbalances active outflux, and a steady-state limiting gradient is established.

Given the great permeability of the descending limb to water, there is a net diffusion of water[1] out of the descending limb and into the interstitium until the osmolarities are equal. The interstitial osmolarity is maintained at 400 mOsm/liter during this equilibration because of continued sodium chloride transport out of the ascending limb.

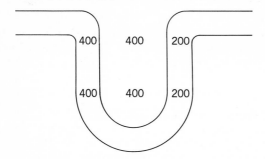

Note that the osmolarities of the descending limb and interstitium are equal and both are higher than that of the ascending limb. So far we have held the fluid stationary in the loop, but, of course, it is actually continuously flowing. Let us look at what occurs under conditions of flow. We shall simplify the analysis by assuming that flow through the loop, on the one hand, and ion and water movements, on the other, occur in discontinuous, out-of-phase steps. During the stationary phase, as described above, sodium chloride is transported out of the ascending limb to establish a gradient of 200 mOsm/liter, and water diffuses out of

---

[1] The descending limb is not completely impermeable to sodium and chloride. Accordingly, some of these ions diffuse into the loop simultaneously with water movement out of the loop. For simplicity, we ignore this additional complexity. (See Kokko, 1974, in Suggested Readings for Chap. 5.)

the descending limb until descending limb and interstitium have the same osmolarity. During the flow phase, fluid leaves the loop via the distal tubule, and new fluid enters the loop from the proximal tubule (Fig. 11).

Note that the fluid is progressively concentrated as it flows down the descending limb and then is progressively diluted as it flows up the ascending limb. While only a 200 mOsm/liter gradient is maintained across the ascending limb at any giving *horizontal level* in the medulla, there exists a much larger osmotic gradient from the top of the medulla to the bottom (312 mOsm/liter versus 700 mOsm/liter). In other words, the 200 mOsm/liter gradient established by active (sodium) chloride transport has been *multiplied* because of the *countercurrent* flow (i.e., flow in opposing directions through the two limbs of a loop) within the loop. It should be emphasized that the active-chloride-transport mechanism within the ascending limb is the essential component of the entire system; without it, the countercurrent flow would have no effect whatsoever on concentrations.

The highest concentration achieved at the tip of the loop depends upon many factors, particularly the length of the loop (the kangaroo rat has extremely long loops) and the strength of the chloride pump. In humans, the value reached is 1,400 mOsm/liter, which, you will recall, is also the maximal concentration of the excreted urine. But what has this system really accomplished? Certainly, it concentrates the loop fluid to 1,400 mOsm/liter, but then it immediately redilutes the fluid so that the fluid entering the distal tubule is actually more dilute than the plasma. Where is the *final urine* concentrated and how?

The site of final concentration is in the collecting ducts. Recall that the collecting ducts course through the renal medulla, parallel to the loops of Henle, and are bathed by the interstitial fluid of the medulla. As described above, in the presence of maximal levels of ADH, fluid leaves the distal tubules isoosmotic to plasma, i.e., at 300 mOsm/liter. As this fluid flows through the collecting ducts, it equilibrates with the ever-increasing osmolarity of the interstitial fluid. Thus, the real function of the loop countercurrent multiplier system is to concentrate the *medullary interstitium*. Under the influence of ADH, the collecting ducts are highly permeable to water, which diffuses out of the collecting ducts and into the interstitium as a result of the osmotic gradient (Fig. 12). The net result is that the fluid at the end of the collecting duct has equilibrated with the interstitial fluid at the tip of the medulla. In the presence of low plasma-ADH concentrations, the collecting ducts, like the distal tubules, become relatively impermeable to water, and the interstitial osmotic gradient is ineffective in inducing water movement out of the collecting ducts.

Let us summarize the overall net movement of sodium chloride and

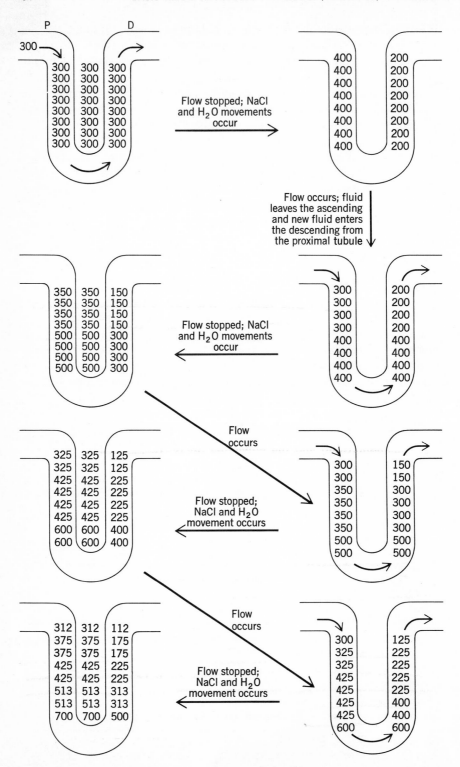

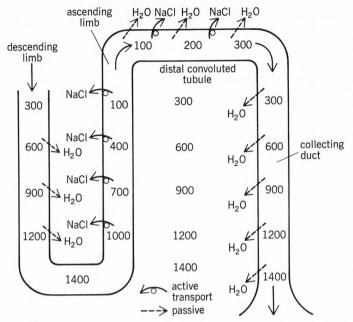

Figure 12 Interactions of loop of Henle and collecting duct in formation of a concentrated urine (see footnotes, pages 52 and 55).

water out of the tubules and into the medullary interstitium during formation of a concentrated urine. First, sodium chloride is lost from the ascending limb by active transport of the chloride and passive following by the sodium.[1] This sodium chloride causes net diffusion of water out of the descending limb and the collecting ducts. In the steady state, this sodium chloride and water entering the medullary interstitium must be taken up by capillaries and carried away. This is, of course, the final step during reabsorption of fluid anywhere in the tubules, and it occurs as a result of the usual hydrostatic and colloid osmotic forces acting across the capillary wall.

Countercurrent Exchange: Vasa Recta

There is, however, a unique characteristic of the medullary circulation without which the entire system could not operate, namely, the hairpin-loop anatomy of the medullary vessels (the *vasa recta*), which run paral-

---

[1] As described earlier, sodium is also actively reabsorbed from the collecting ducts. This phenomenon helps to reduce the amount of salt lost to the urine. But it has been ignored in our analysis because it is not an important component of the countercurrent system. (See Giebisch and Windhager, 1973, in Suggested Readings for Chap. 5.)

Figure 11 Countercurrent multiplier system in loop of Henle. (*Redrawn from R. F. Pitts, "Physiology of the Kidney and Body Fluids," 3d ed., Year Book, Chicago, 1974.*)

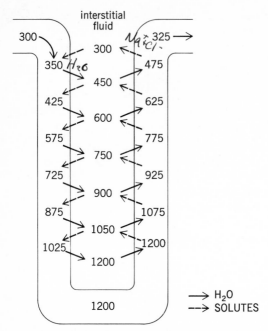

Figure 13 Vasa recta as countercurrent exchangers. (*Redrawn from R. F. Pitts, "Physiology of the Kidney and Body Fluids," 3d ed., Year Book, Chicago, 1974.*)

lel to the loops of Henle and collecting ducts (Fig. 3). The problem is this: What would happen to the medullary gradient if the medulla were supplied with ordinary (as opposed to hairpin-loop) capillaries? As plasma having the usual osmolarity of 300 mOsm/liter entered the highly concentrated environment of the medulla, there would be massive net diffusion of sodium chloride into the capillaries and of water out of the capillaries. Thus the interstitial gradient would soon be lost. But, with hairpin loops, the sequence of events shown in Fig. 13 occurs. Blood enters the capillary loop at an osmolarity of 300 mOsm/liter, and as it flows down the capillary loop deeper and deeper into the medulla, sodium chloride does indeed diffuse into, and water out of, the capillary. However, after the bend in the loop is reached, the blood then flows up the ascending capillary loop, where the process is almost completely reversed. Thus the capillary loop is acting as a so-called *countercurrent exchanger,* which prevents the gradient from being dissipated. Note that the capillary is, itself, completely passive; i.e., it is not *creating* the medullary gradient, only protecting it. Its passive nature explains why it is called an exchanger; compare its function to that of the loop of Henle, which actively creates the gradient and is therefore a multiplier. Finally, it should be noted that the hairpin-loop structure essentially eliminates losses, by *diffusion,* of solute or water from the interstitium. It does not, though, prevent the *bulk flow* of medullary interstitial fluid into the vasa recta secondary to the usual Starling forces. By this bulk-flow process, the net salt and water entering the interstitium from the loops and collecting ducts is carried away, and the steady-state gradient is maintained.

The above description of the countercurrent multiplier system for urinary concentration underestimates the complexity of the overall operation. A major ignored complexity is the fact that the thin portion of the ascending loop of Henle may function differently from the thick portion (see footnote, page 51). A second factor of great importance is urea. In very important ways urea participates in determining maximal concentrating ability. Indeed, of the 1,400 mOsm in a liter of urine, almost half of this is urea, and much of the medullary gradient is made up of urea. Other ions, too, play at least minor roles. However, we have chosen not to discuss these other complex variables but to focus attention on the absolutely essential factors, namely, the interactions between sodium chloride and water movements in the loops of Henle, collecting ducts, and vasa recta. The interested reader should consult the Suggested Readings listed at the back.

A point of considerable clinical importance is that inability to achieve maximal urinary concentration occurs early in any renal disease because of interference with the establishment of the medullary gradient. Any significant change in renal structure, particularly in the medulla, can upset the intricate geometric relationships required for maximal countercurrent functioning. A change in renal blood flow to the medulla, either too much or too little, will reduce the gradient by carrying away too much or too little water and/or solute. Destruction of the loops will also reduce the gradient, as will decreased chloride pumping by the ascending limb. The latter may be caused by tubular disease or by a marked reduction in GFR and, thereby, a reduction in the supply of chloride to the loop.

Finally, it should be emphasized that, although the entire discussion of renal concentrating ability has been in terms of urine osmolarity, the usual clinical measurement of urine "concentration" is *specific gravity*. The determination of specific gravity requires only a hydrometer and is easy and cheap to perform. However, specific gravity is really a measure of urine density, not of concentration. Frequently, the two correlate well, but under certain circumstances they can be quite divergent, since specific gravity is influenced by the nature as well as by the number of solute particles. For example, protein in the urine causes the specific gravity to be increased with little change in osmolarity.

SUMMARY

Figure 14 summarizes the previously described changes in volume and osmolarity of the tubular fluid as it flows along the nephron.

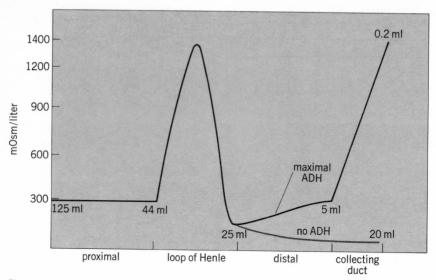

Figure 14 Changes in volume and osmolarity of the tubular fluid as it flows along the nephron.

1   Approximately 65 percent of the filtered water and sodium chloride are reabsorbed in the proximal tubule, but the fluid remains isoosmotic.

2   In the loop, water is reabsorbed from the descending limb, but much more sodium chloride is reabsorbed from the ascending limb so that hypoosmotic fluid enters the distal tubule.

3   Only from the distal tubule on does the presence or absence of ADH matter.

4   With essentially no ADH, very little water is reabsorbed from the distal tubule and collecting duct. Consequently, a large volume of dilute urine is formed.

5   With maximal ADH, water reabsorption is high in the distal tubule and collecting ducts. By the end of the distal tubule the fluid has once more become isoosmotic. Almost all the remaining water is reabsorbed in the collecting duct, and a tiny volume of highly concentrated urine is formed.

Several other points of great importance should be reemphasized: (1) Excretion of large quantities of sodium *always* results in the excretion of large quantities of water. This follows from the passive nature of water reabsorption, since water can be reabsorbed only if sodium is reabsorbed first. As we shall see, this relationship has considerable importance for the regulation of extracellular volume. (2) In contrast, large quantities of water can be excreted even though the urine is virtually free of sodium, since a decreased ADH will increase water excretion without altering sodium transport. This process we shall find crucial for the renal regulation of extracellular osmolarity.

Given the basic renal processes for handling sodium, chloride, and water, we now turn to the mechanisms by which they are controlled so as to homeostatically regulate salt and water balance.

Study questions: **15** to **21**

Chapter 6

Control of Sodium and Water Excretion: Regulation of Extracellular Volume and Osmolarity

OBJECTIVES

The student understands the renal regulation of extracellular volume and osmolarity.

1 States the formula relating the filtration, reabsorption, and excretion of sodium
2 Describes the probable nature and locations of "sodium" receptors in the body
3 Lists the efferent inputs controlling GFR and how these inputs change as a result of changes in sodium balance or fluid volumes
4 Defines glomerulotubular balance and describes its significance
5 States the origin of aldosterone, its sites of action, and its effects
6 Defines third factor and lists its probable components
7 Describes peritubular-capillary dynamics and how these physical factors influence sodium reabsorption; states how changes in filtration fraction influence sodium reabsorption; predicts the changes in physical factors which occur with changes in sodium or fluid balance and how they alter sodium and water reabsorption
8 Defines redistribution of blood flow and states how it might influence sodium and water excretion

 9 Lists the factors controlling aldosterone secretion and states which is most important
10 Describes the renin-angiotensin system and the control of renin secretion; lists the biological effects of angiotensin
11 Distinguishes between primary and secondary hyperaldosteronism; describes the hormonal changes in each and the presence or absence of escape
12 Describes the origin of ADH, the reflex controls of its secretion, and its sites of action; defines diabetes insipidus
13 Distinguishes between the reflex changes which occur when an individual has suffered fluid loss because of diarrhea as opposed to a pure water loss, i.e., solute-water loss as opposed to pure-water loss
14 Calculates the changes in body-fluid volumes and osmolarity resulting from the excretion of a known volume of urine having a given osmolarity
15 Describes the control of thirst
16 Diagrams in flow-sheet form the pathways by which sodium and water excretion are altered in response to sweating, diarrhea, hemorrhage, high or low salt diet

Since sodium is freely filterable at the glomerulus and actively reabsorbed but not secreted by the tubules, the amount of sodium excreted in the final urine represents the results of two processes, glomerular filtration and tubular reabsorption:

$$\text{Sodium excretion} = \text{sodium filtered} - \text{sodium reabsorbed}$$
$$= (\text{GFR} \times P_{\text{Na}}) - \text{sodium reabsorbed}$$

It is possible, therefore, to adjust sodium excretion by controlling any of these three variables (Fig. 15). In fact, P_{Na} generally shows little variation, and the reflex control of GFR and sodium reabsorption predominate. For example, what happens if the quantity of filtered sodium increases as a result of a higher GFR but the rate of reabsorption remains constant? Clearly, sodium excretion increases. The same final result could be achieved by lowering sodium reabsorption while the GFR remains constant. Finally, sodium excretion could be raised greatly by elevating the GFR and simultaneously reducing reabsorption. Conversely, sodium excretion could be decreased below normal levels by lowering the GFR or by raising sodium reabsorption, or by both.

The reflex pathways by which changes in total body sodium balance lead to changes in GFR and sodium reabsorption include: (1) "sodium" receptors and the afferent pathways leading from them to the central nervous system and endocrine glands; (2) efferent neural and hormonal pathways to the kidneys; and (3) renal effector sites i.e., the renal arterioles and tubules.

The first component of the reflexes, the so-called sodium receptors,

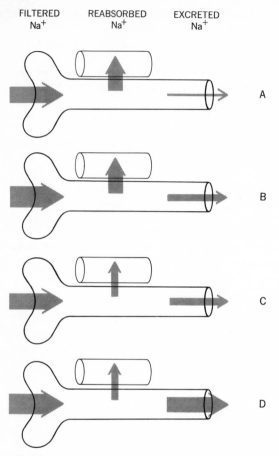

Figure 15 Sodium excretion is increased by increasing the GFR (B), by decreasing reabsorption (C), or by a combination of both (D). The arrows indicate relative magnitudes of filtration, reabsorption, and excretion. (*From A. J. Vander et al., "Human Physiology," © 1970 by McGraw-Hill, Inc. Used with permission of McGraw-Hill Book Company.*)

offers considerable theoretical difficulties. There is no way that the total body *mass* of sodium can be detected by any imaginable receptor. Therefore, one must look for some other variable which correlates closely with total body sodium and which might constitute the critical signal. As shown in the following examples, the ideal candidate is the volume of extracellular fluid.

What happens, for example, when a person ingests a liter of isotonic sodium chloride, i.e., a solution of salt with exactly the same osmolarity as the body fluids? It is absorbed from the gastrointestinal tract into the plasma, from which most of it then enters the interstitial fluid. The important fact is that all the salt and water remain in the extracellular fluid (plasma and interstitial fluid) and none enters the cells. Because of the active sodium pumps in cell membranes, sodium is effectively barred from the cells. The water, too, remains, since only the volume and not the osmolarity of the extracellular compartment has been changed; i.e., no osmotic gradient exists to drive the ingested water into cells.

Another example: A man ingests 145 mmol of sodium chloride but no water. The salt is distributed in the extracellular fluid but is barred from the cells. The addition of this water-free solute to the extracellular fluid causes extracellular osmolarity to rise above intracellular osmolarity; therefore, water diffuses out of the cells and into the extracellular fluid until the osmolarities are once more equal. The net result is an expansion of extracellular volume and a decrease of intracellular volume.

These examples lead us to the extremely important generalization that the total extracellular-fluid volume depends primarily upon the mass of extracellular sodium, which, in turn, correlates directly with total body sodium, since sodium is effectively barred from cells. (There are considerable amounts of sodium in bone, but this fact does not seriously alter the analysis.) It should now be clear why reflexes which maintain extracellular volume constant simultaneously keep total body sodium constant.

Yet, how can there be receptors capable of detecting changes in the total extracellular volume? The answer is almost certainly that there are not any and that total extracellular volume, per se, is also not *directly* monitored. What about its component volumes—plasma volume and interstitial volume? Again it seems unlikely that either of these is *directly* monitored. What seems most likely at present is that closely correlated derivative functions of these volumes, i.e., *intravascular* and *intracardiac pressures, cardiac output,* and *organ blood flow,* are the actual variables monitored. Thus, a decrease in plasma volume generally tends to lower the hydrostatic pressures within the veins, cardiac chambers, and arteries. These changes are detected by baroreceptors within the blood vessels, e.g., the carotid sinus, and within the cardiac chambers. Such baroreceptors undoubtedly constitute much of the important input for regulation of sodium excretion. Other derivatives of plasma volume are cardiac output (decreased volume → decreased atrial pressure → decreased output) and, in turn, blood flow through various organs. It is likely that these variables, too, are monitored and reflexly induce changes in sodium excretion. There are probably additional variables also dependent on extracellular volume which take part in the reflexes. At present, it is not possible to assign quantitative roles to specific receptors.

In summary, then, regulation of total body sodium and extracellular volume depends not upon sodium or volume receptors but rather upon

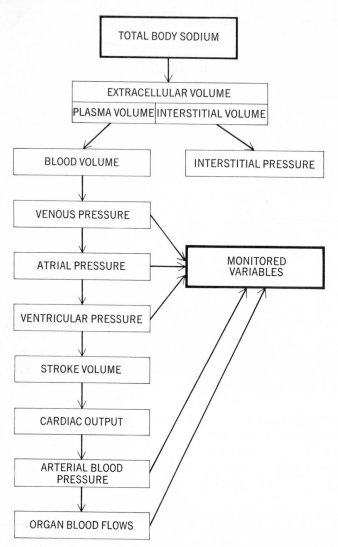

Figure 16   Flow sheet demonstrating the series of derivative variables dependent upon total body sodium. In no case is any block in the sequence totally dependent upon the previous one, for other factors are also involved. The major aim of the figure is to demonstrate how a change in body sodium could result in changes in a group of monitored variables which could be detected by receptors and initiate the responses controlling sodium excretion.

pressure, distention, or flow receptors in various parts of the body (see Fig. 16). In the normal person, regulation of these variables results in excellent homeostasis of body sodium and extracellular-fluid volume, since these parameters are all so dependent upon one another. However, as we shall see, disease states can produce striking discrepancies between them with a resulting abnormal expansion of extracellular volume and total body sodium.

CONTROL OF GFR

We have described the three factors which determine the GFR: glomerular-capillary blood pressure, Bowman's capsule hydrostatic pressure, and plasma protein concentration (i.e., plasma colloid osmotic pressure). Anything which alters the magnitude of these factors can be expected to change the GFR. Physiologically, the GFR is controlled primarily by the alteration both of glomerular-capillary pressure and of plasma protein concentration.

Physiological Regulation of Glomerular-Capillary Pressure

(1) A fall in arterial blood pressure decreases filtration rate by lowering glomerular-capillary pressure. Conversely, an increase in arterial blood pressure has just the opposite effect. Recall, however, that, because of renal autoregulation, arterial-pressure changes, per se, have only small effects on GFR over the usual physiological range. On the other hand, any large decrease in arterial pressure definitely would significantly reduce glomerular-capillary pressure and, thereby, GFR.

(2) A decrease in the diameter of the afferent arterioles, secondary to increased renal sympathetic activity or circulating epinephrine, lowers glomerular-capillary pressure and filtration rate because a larger fraction of the arterial pressure is dissipated in overcoming the increased resistance offered by the narrowed arterioles. These sympathetic pathways play prominent roles in the reflexes which regulate arterial blood pressure, being activated by a lowered blood pressure and inhibited by an elevated pressure. To take a specific example: What changes in renal hemodynamics occur as a result of severe salt and water loss due to diarrhea (Fig. 17)? The decreased plasma volume resulting from salt and water loss prevents adequate venous return, thereby reducing atrial pressure, cardiac output, and arterial blood pressure. These drops in blood pressure are detected by the carotid sinuses and aortic arch, as well as by other baroreceptors in the veins and atria. The information is relayed to the medullary cardiovascular centers, which respond by inhibiting parasympathetic outflow to the heart and by stimulating sympathetic outflow to the heart and to arteriolar smooth muscle. The sympathetic stimulation of the renal arterioles (both by the renal nerves and by epinephrine from the adrenal medulla) increases constriction of the renal arterioles. This vasoconstriction increases the resistance to blood flow from the renal artery to the glomerular capillaries, lowering the capillary blood pressure and GFR. By this mechanism, both the amount of

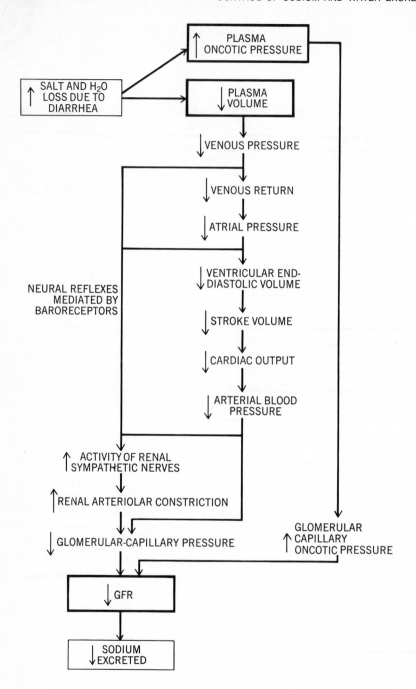

sodium filtered and the amount of sodium excreted are reduced, and further loss from the body is prevented. Conversely, an increased GFR can result from greater plasma volume and contribute to the increased renal sodium loss which returns extracellular volume to normal. This analysis is in terms of a logical stimulus for GFR control, namely, changes in blood pressure, but the sympathetic outflow via the medullary cardiovascular center can be changed in response to a variety of stimuli, such as pain, fright, and exercise; accordingly, fluid excretion may be altered at least transiently by many situations.

In this and subsequent discussions we emphasize the significance of the sympathetic nervous system as a major efferent pathway for GFR regulation. As noted earlier, the renal arterioles are also sensitive to a variety of humoral agents, such as prostaglandins and histamine, which *may* function as efferent inputs. However, although it seems almost certain that one or more of these agents does play a significant role, their specific contributions and the reflex pathways controlling them are undetermined at present.

Physiological Changes in Plasma Protein Concentration

There are frequent situations in which changes in plasma or extracellular volume are associated with changes in plasma protein concentration. In such situations, changes in colloid osmotic pressure may also play an important role in the physiological raising or lowering of GFR. For example, the severe fluid loss of sweating or diarrhea will lower the extracellular volume, but at the same time it will concentrate plasma protein. The resulting increase in colloid osmotic pressure will reduce net filtration pressure in the glomeruli and, thereby, GFR. Conversely, a marked increase in salt uptake will increase extracellular volume and, at least transiently, lower plasma protein concentration. The result is lowered colloid osmotic pressure and increased GFR.

In each of these examples, the change in plasma protein concentration is in the appropriate direction to reestablish salt balance by decreasing or increasing salt excretion. Is this also true for hemorrhage? The answer is *no*. Hemorrhage, per se, does not immediately alter plasma protein concentration since all blood components are lost in *equivalent* proportions. However, the blood loss is followed by a net

Figure 17 Pathway by which the GFR is decreased when plasma volume decreases. The baroreceptors which initiate the sympathetic reflex are probably located in large veins and in the walls of the heart, as well as in the carotid sinuses and aortic arch. There may be important efferent inputs other than the sympathetic neurons, but they have not been clearly established. (*Modified from A. J. Vander et al., "Human Physiology,"* © *1970 by McGraw-Hill, Inc. Used with permission of McGraw-Hill Book Company.*)

movement of interstitial fluid into the vascular compartment. This entry of protein-free fluid lowers the plasma protein concentration and tends to raise GFR—an inappropriate response, since sodium conservation, not increased sodium loss, is the "desired" response to hemorrhage. However, GFR does decrease in response to hemorrhage, despite the fact that colloid osmotic pressure is going in the wrong direction. Why? Because decreased arterial pressure and reflexly increased sympathetic outflow to the afferent arterioles cause glomerular-capillary pressure to fall by a larger amount than colloid osmotic pressure falls.[1] This example is presented as a reminder of the fact that renal responses to any given situation represent the algebraic sum of multiple inputs.

CONTROL OF TUBULAR SODIUM REABSORPTION

Present evidence indicates that, so far as long-term regulation of sodium excretion is concerned, the control of tubular sodium reabsorption is probably more important than that of GFR (even though, as we shall see, the former is somewhat dependent on the latter). For example, patients with chronic marked reductions of GFR usually maintain normal sodium excretion by decreasing tubular sodium reabsorption.

Glomerulotubular Balance   Reabsorp varies ⊂ GFR

One reason for the lesser importance of changes in the filtered load of sodium is the fact that the reabsorption of fluid in the proximal tubules, and probably the loops of Henle, as well, varies directly with glomerular filtration rate. This phenomenon is known as *glomerulotubular balance.* For example, if GFR is experimentally decreased by 25 percent, the rate of proximal fluid reabsorption is observed to decrease by almost the same amount, perhaps by 20 percent. The mechanisms responsible for automatically adjusting tubular reabsorption to GFR are not clear. It is certain, however, that they are completely intrarenal; i.e., glomerulotubular balance requires no external neural or hormonal input and can be shown to occur in a completely isolated kidney. The net effect of this phenomenon is to *blunt* the ability of GFR changes per se to produce *large* changes in sodium excretion. However, for several reasons, it is incorrect to assume that, because of glomerulotubular balance, sodium excretion is *completely* unaffected by changes in filtered load. First, glomerulotubular balance is not absolute; i.e., the changes in reabsorption and GFR are not usually exactly proportional. Second, this phenomenon is limited primarily to the proximal tubules and to the loops of Henle. The proper conclusion is that changes in the filtered load of sodium do, per se, result in changes in sodium excretion, but the changes are greatly mitigated by glomerulotubular balance.

[1] Deen et al., 1974 (Suggested Readings) describe another control of glomerular COP.

Like autoregulation of blood flow, glomerulotubular balance is an inherent renal process requiring no nerves or hormones external to the kidney. In a sense, glomerulotubular balance is a second line of defense preventing any spontaneous changes in GFR, such as occur after a large protein meal, from causing large changes in sodium excretion. The first line of defense is GFR autoregulation. In other words, autoregulation prevents GFR from changing too much in response to spontaneous changes in blood pressure, and glomerulotubular balance blunts the sodium-excretion response to whatever GFR change does occur. This allows major responsibility for control of sodium excretion to reside in those factors to be described next—aldosterone and so-called third factor.

Aldosterone

Control of Na⁺ Excretion

A major clue to the control of sodium reabsorption was the observation that patients whose adrenal glands are diseased or missing excrete large quantities of sodium in the urine. Indeed, if untreated, they may die because of low blood pressure resulting from depletion of plasma volume. This increased sodium excretion often occurs despite lowered GFR, thus establishing that decreased tubular reabsorption is the factor responsible for the sodium loss. The adrenal influence on sodium reabsorption is mediated by a hormone, *aldosterone,* produced by the *adrenal cortex,* specifically in the cortical area known as the *zona glomerulosa.* (This term is somewhat unfortunate because it sounds like a description of a kidney area rather than of an adrenal zone.) Aldosterone stimulates sodium reabsorption primarily in the distal tubules and collecting ducts. The total quantity of sodium reabsorption dependent upon the influence of aldosterone is approximately 2 percent of the total filtered sodium. Thus, in the complete absence of aldosterone, one would excrete 2 percent of the filtered sodium; whereas, in the presence of maximal plasma concentrations of aldosterone, virtually no sodium would be excreted. Two percent of the filtered sodium may, at first thought, seem small, but it is actually very large because of the huge volume of glomerular filtrate:

$$\text{Total filtered NaCl/day} = \text{GFR} \times P_{\text{NaCl}}$$
$$= 180 \text{ liters/day} \times 9 \text{ gm/liter}$$
$$= 1,620 \text{ gm/day}$$

Thus, aldosterone controls the reabsorption of $0.02 \times 1,620$ gm/day = 33.4 gm/day, an amount considerably more than the average person eats. Therefore, by reflex variation of plasma concentrations of aldosterone between minimal and maximal, the excretion of sodium can be finely adjusted to the intake so that total body sodium and extracellular volume remain constant.

It is interesting that aldosterone also stimulates sodium transport by other epithelia in the body, namely, by sweat and salivary glands and by the intestine. The net effect is the same as that exerted on the kidney — a reduction in the sodium content of the luminal fluid. Thus, aldosterone is an all-purpose stimulator of sodium retention. This hormone, like other steroids, exerts its effect by stimulating RNA synthesis, but the manner in which this event is coupled to increased sodium transport is far from settled. The control of aldosterone secretion is described after the section on third factor.

② Third Factor

Until recently, most renal physiologists believed that the control of sodium excretion could be explained completely in terms of changes in GFR and in aldosterone-dependent tubular sodium reabsorption. It is now clear that these two factors do not suffice and that there must exist a third factor which influences sodium reabsorption.

The term *third factor* was coined before much information was available concerning its identity. It is now clear that the moiety of sodium reabsorption not controlled by aldosterone is regulated not by just one third factor but by a variety of inputs. They are still lumped together as third factor — in large part because the precise contributions of each is still not clear. The inputs are natriuretic hormone, physical factors, and redistribution of renal blood flow.

Natriuretic Hormone The evidence for the existence of a *natriuretic,* or salt-losing hormone, is highly controversial. Some evidence suggests that such a hormone exists and that it is released when extracellular volume is expanded (e.g., by saline infusions), but little more can be said with certainty at this time.

Physical Factors There is now general agreement that intrarenal *physical factors* are a major component of third factor. It was largely in anticipation of this discussion that we described the separate steps involved in fluid reabsorption — specifically the fact that, although active sodium (or chloride) transport is the key event in salt and water reabsorption, the final step is the bulk flow of fluid from the interstitial space into the peritubular capillaries. The forces which determine this flow are the same as for any capillary — the hydrostatic and oncotic, or colloid osmotic, pressure differences acting across the capillary:

Net pressure for fluid movement into peritubular capillaries
$$= P_{Int} + \pi_{PC} - P_{PC} - \pi_{Int}$$

where the subscripts Int and PC stand for interstitium and peritubular capillary, respectively.

This is the second time we have dealt with capillary dynamics in the kidney, the first being the discussion of glomerular filtration. It must be emphasized that the concepts are identical, but, of course, the locations are different. Glomerular dynamics involve the balance of forces between the glomerular capillaries and Bowman's capsule; whereas the peritubular forces are between the interstitium and the peritubular capillaries. Whereas the net driving pressure across the glomeruli always favors filtration out of the capillaries into Bowman's capsule, the net driving pressure across the peritubular capillaries always favors net movement into the capillaries (reabsorption). The major reason for the latter fact is twofold: (1) the peritubular-capillary hydrostatic pressure is generally quite low (10 to 15 mmHg) because the blood entering the peritubular capillaries has already had to flow through the afferent arterioles, glomeruli, and efferent arterioles. (2) The oncotic pressure of the plasma entering the peritubular capillaries is higher than that of the plasma entering the glomeruli. The former has had its proteins concentrated by loss of protein-free filtrate during passage through the glomerular capillaries. (Early peritubular-capillary oncotic pressure is, therefore, identical to end-glomerular-capillary oncotic pressure.)

Since bulk flow into the peritubular capillaries is the final step in tubular fluid reabsorption, it should not be too surprising that any reduction in the net driving pressure favoring this final step causes a decreased tubular net salt and water reabsorption; the converse is also true. Thus increased hydrostatic pressure in the peritubular capillaries (resulting either from an increased arterial blood pressure or from renal arteriolar vasodilation) inhibits fluid reabsorption. Conversely, decreased arterial pressure or renal vasoconstriction is associated with increased reabsorption. Changes in the oncotic pressure of the plasma in the peritubular capillaries also influence fluid reabsorption. As would be predicted, an increased oncotic pressure facilitates reabsorption, whereas a decreased oncotic pressure reduces reabsorption. Thus, in the previous section we saw that changes in *glomerular-capillary* hydrostatic and oncotic pressures were controlled so as to regulate GFR and, thereby, sodium excretion, and now we see that analogous changes in the *peritubular-capillary* hydrostatic and oncotic pressures regulate sodium reabsorption and, thereby, sodium excretion.

Teleologically, it makes good sense that such changes in these physical factors regulate sodium balance and extracellular volume by altering sodium reabsorption. Volume depletion (as in our example of diarrhea) causes decreased peritubular-capillary hydrostatic pressure (just as it does decreased glomerular-capillary hydrostatic pressure) because of reduced arterial pressure and reflex renal vasoconstriction (Fig. 18). The effect of the reduced pressure is to enhance sodium reabsorption. The sodium depletion also causes concentration of plasma protein, and this increased oncotic pressure also enhances tubular sodium reabsorption, just as it reduces GFR.

In the last example above, the change in peritubular-capillary on-

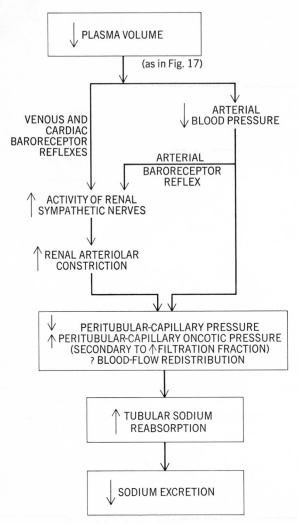

Figure 18 Pathway by which changes in intrarenal physical factors and blood-flow redistribution are elicited by changes in plasma volume. Compare this to the figure for GFR control; clearly the same inputs that tend to lower GFR also tend to increase sodium reabsorption. Again it should be noted that as yet unidentified hormonal factors may also serve, along with the sympathetic nervous system, as important efferent inputs to the renal arterioles.

cotic pressure simply reflects a change in systemic plasma oncotic pressure. Now, we introduce a new but predictable fact: Peritubular-capillary oncotic pressure can be changed independently of any changes in systemic oncotic pressure. The facts needed to understand this phenomenon have already been given: Peritubular-capillary oncotic pressure *always* differs from systemic oncotic pressure, since the plasma proteins are concentrated by loss of protein-free filtrate during passage through the glomerular capillaries. The degree of oncotic-pressure increase depends upon the fraction of the renal plasma flow which is filtered at the glomerulus; this *filtration fraction* is not always the same but varies depending upon the distribution of renal arteriolar constriction. Recall that reflex vasoconstriction mediated either by the renal nerves or by circulating agents generally affects not only the afferent arterioles but the efferent as well, though to a lesser degree. The net result is a greater reduction in renal blood flow than in GFR, i.e., an increased filtration fraction, a larger-than-normal increase in peritubular-capillary oncotic pressure, and an increased reabsorption of sodium. Conversely, reflexly induced renal vasodilation (as might occur after increased ingestion of salt and water) would be associated with a decreased filtration fraction, a smaller-than-normal rise in peritubular-capillary oncotic pressure, and less sodium reabsorption. Thus, filtration fraction, by altering peritubular-capillary oncotic pressure, is an important determinant of sodium reabsorption.

Intuitively, it may seem obvious that the rate of sodium reabsorption depends upon these Starling forces, since they are responsible for the last step in the overall process, the movement of fluid from the interstitium into the capillary. On the other hand, it might also seem intuitively likely that the active component of sodium transport should somehow be able to compensate for this. The fact is that the active transport of sodium *into the intercellular spaces* may very well continue at an unchanged rate, but the Starling forces determine how much of this salt and water actually goes on into the capillary rather than simply leaking back into the tubular lumen. The sequence is probably as follows: An increase in peritubular-capillary hydrostatic pressure or a decrease in oncotic pressure retards fluid movement from the intercellular spaces into the capillary. As active salt transport and passive water movement out of the tubular lumen continues, fluid accumulates in the intercellular spaces, causing the tissue to swell. This change in dimensions or pressure loosens the tight junctions between the tubular cells; therefore, an increased fraction of the intercellular sodium chloride and water leaks back into the tubular lumen rather than continuing on into the capillaries. Thus, the *net reabsorption* (movement of fluid from tubular lumen into capillary) is decreased.

Redistribution of Blood Flow Another potential mechanism for altering sodium excretion is the type of *redistribution of blood flow* described earlier. Present data suggest that nephrons in the superficial cortex may have less capacity to reabsorb sodium than do nephrons in the juxtamedullary cortex. Were this true, then at any given total GFR, the relative amounts of fluid filtered by the two different nephron populations would be an important determinant of sodium excretion. Specifically, a redistribution of flow to the inner cortex, secondary, say, to increased sympathetic input to the outer cortex (Fig. 18) would be associated with decreased sodium excretion because of the greater capacity of these nephrons to reabsorb sodium. A definite answer is not yet available, but this may well be an important reflex mechanism for control of sodium balance.

Other Known Hormones

Cortisol, estrogen, growth hormone, and several other known hormones may influence sodium excretion under certain conditions. However, there is no reason to believe that these factors, like the ones described above, are reflexly controlled so as to homeostatically regulate sodium balance.

CONTROL OF ALDOSTERONE SECRETION

How is aldosterone secretion controlled? At least four distinct inputs to the adrenal gland are recognized at present: (1) plasma sodium concentration, (2) plasma potassium concentration, (3) adrenocorticotropic hormone (ACTH), and (4) angiotensin.

The first two of these inputs are not mediated by nerves or by hormones. Rather, the adrenal cortex responds to the sodium and potassium concentrations of the blood perfusing it or to some adrenal intracellular derivative of these concentrations, such as adrenal-cell sodium concentration. The fact that aldosterone secretion is controlled, in part, by plasma sodium concentration makes good sense: Increased plasma sodium → decreased aldosterone secretion → decreased tubular sodium reabsorption → increased sodium excretion → decreased plasma sodium concentration. However, in man, this is only a minor control of aldosterone secretion—a fact which also makes sense teleologically, since plasma sodium *concentration* generally changes very little despite marked changes in extracellular *volume*. (Remember that water movements into or out of body cells tend to keep osmolarity and, thereby, plasma sodium concentration, relatively stable.) The influence of plasma potassium concentration on aldosterone secretion is important and will be described in the section on renal handling of potassium.

ACTH is the hormone from the anterior pituitary which controls secretion of the other major adrenocortical hormone, cortisol. There is no question that, when ACTH is secreted in very large amounts, it also stimulates aldosterone secretion. However, the relationship of ACTH to sodium homeostasis is not of primary importance.

We are left with our fourth input, angiotensin, as the most important known controller of aldosterone secretion in sodium-regulating reflexes. What is the origin of angiotensin, and what controls its blood level? In order to answer these questions, we must describe the overall *renin-angiotensin hormonal system.*

RENIN-ANGIOTENSIN SYSTEM

Basic Components

Renin is a proteolytic enzyme secreted into the blood by the kidneys, specifically by the specialized area of each nephron known as the *juxtaglomerular (JG) apparatus* (Fig. 19). Each JG apparatus is composed of three anatomical structures: (1) *granular, or juxtaglomerular, cells;* (2) *the macula densa;* and (3) connective-tissue cells. The granular cells appear to be differentiated smooth muscle cells in the walls of the arterioles (particularly in the afferent arterioles) where the arterioles junction with the glomeruli. The granular cells secrete renin. The macula densa is the specialized portion of tubule that marks the transition from the ascending loop of Henle to the distal tubule. This nephron segment always touches the afferent arteriole and glomerulus from its own nephron of origin, and the macula densa cells, themselves, are in intimate contact with the granular cells. Evidence suggests that the macula densa contributes to the control of renin secretion. Once in the bloodstream, renin catalyzes the splitting of a decapeptide, *angiotensin I,* from a protein in plasma known as *angiotensinogen* (Fig. 20). Under the influence of another enzyme, *converting enzyme,* two amino acids are

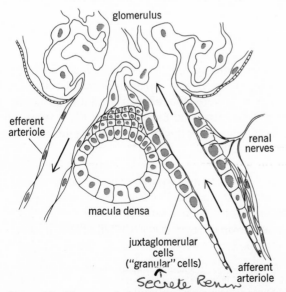

Figure 19   Diagram of glomerulus showing the juxtaglomerular apparatus. [*Redrawn from J. O. Davis,* Amer. J. Med., **55:**333 (1973).]

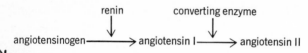

Figure 20 Formation of angiotensin II in the blood. Renin is normally rate-limiting.

then split from the relatively inactive angiotensin I to yield the active octapeptide, *angiotensin II*. Angiotensin II is usually referred to simply as angiotensin.

Angiotensin has many biological effects. It is perhaps the most powerful vasoconstrictor known. Not only does it act directly upon *arteriolar* smooth muscle to cause contraction, but it also stimulates (in several ways and at various locations) the outflow of the sympathetic nervous system. Because of these effects, its potential role in hypertension has received much attention. It also acts upon the brain to stimulate thirst, and it may influence other types of behavior. In this section we are concerned with its ability to stimulate the adrenal secretion of aldosterone.

The liver synthesizes and secretes angiotensinogen, which is usually present in the blood in high concentration. The origin of converting enzyme is unclear, and the conversion of angiotensin I to angiotensin II seems to occur mainly as blood flows through the lung capillaries. At any rate, converting enzyme, like angiotensinogen, is usually present in excess; accordingly, the primary determinant of the rate of angiotensin formation is the plasma concentration of renin. Therefore, the critical question becomes: What controls the rate of renin secretion by the kidneys?

Control of Renin Secretion

The answer to this question is quite complex, since there are at least four types of inputs which are, in some ways, strongly interrelated with one another. Indeed it is proving a very difficult task to untangle them. The four mechanisms[1] are (1) an intrarenal baroreceptor, (2) a tubular sodium receptor in the macula densa, (3) the renal sympathetic nerves, and (4) angiotensin itself.

Intrarenal Baroreceptors The renin-secreting granular cells, themselves, may act as baroreceptors (i.e., as pressure or distention receptors) monitoring the pressure or vascular volume within the afferent arterioles and varying their secretion of renin inversely with these param-

---

[1] Present evidence indicates that there are additional inputs (including ADH and potassium) controlling renin release. The interested reader should consult Davis, 1973, and Laragh and Sealey, 1973, in Suggested Readings for Chap. 6.

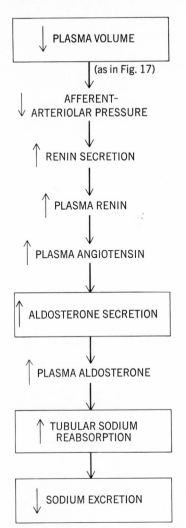

Figure 21 Intrarenal baroreceptor pathway for control of renin release and sodium excretion.

eters. This makes good sense, teleologically. For example, consider the response to diarrhea that was described in the section on control of GFR: The pressure at the ends of the afferent arterioles would be reduced both because of decreased arterial pressure and because of reflexly increased sympathetic outflow to the arterioles (Fig. 21); the decreased arteriolar pressure would cause increased release of renin from the granular cells.

Macula Densa Because of the contact between the granular cells and the macula densa, it is tempting to postulate that the renin-secreting

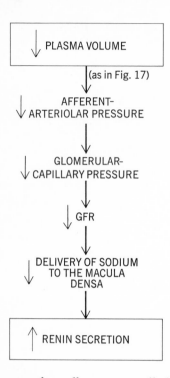

Figure 22 Macula densa pathway for control of renin release. Macula densa sodium load would probably also be reduced because of increased proximal and loop sodium reabsorption (secondary to a change in peritubular physical factors).

granular cells are controlled by input from the macula densa concerning the composition of the early distal-tubular fluid. (Recall that the macula densa is the first portion of the distal tubule.) Experimental evidence suggests that this is the case. Specifically, the evidence suggests that renin secretion is inversely related to the amount of sodium entering the macula densa. Such a reflex also makes sense teleologically, since it is simply a logical extension of the reflex described for the intrarenal-baroreceptor theory (Fig. 22). Indeed, it should be evident why it has been so difficult to distinguish between the baroreceptor and macula densa theories. At present, it seems likely that both types of receptors exist within the kidney and contribute to the control of renin release. In the situation illustrated by Fig. 22, sodium load to the macula densa was decreased because of a reduction in GFR. It should be obvious that macula densa sodium load can also be decreased by increasing proximal and/or loop sodium reabsorption (as, for example, by increasing peritubular oncotic pressure). Finally, it should be pointed out that considerable controversy exists concerning the precise stimulus to the macula densa; we believe the sodium-load story is best supported by present data.

Renal Sympathetic Nerves We have already described one important mechanism by which an increased renal-sympathetic-nerve activity

stimulates renin secretion, namely, by causing constriction of the afferent arterioles. This stimulates the intrarenal baroreceptor by reducing
the hydrostatic pressure at the end of the afferent arteriole, and it also
stimulates the macula densa receptor by reducing GFR and, thereby, the
sodium load to the distal tubule. In this manner, the renal sympathetic
nerves clearly play an important *indirect* role in controlling renin secretion. In addition, sympathetic neurons end in the immediate vicinity of
the granular cells and macula densa, and it seems very likely that these
neurons exert a *direct* stimulatory effect on the JG apparatus via beta-
adrenergic receptors on the cells of the apparatus.

Angiotensin Angiotensin exerts a direct inhibitory effect on renin
secretion by the JG apparatus. This is another example of a negative-
feedback loop in which a hormone inhibits the secretion of its own
stimulating substance analogous to the inhibition of ACTH secretion by
cortisol or to inhibition of TSH secretion by thyroxin. By this mechanism, angiotensin exerts a dampening effect upon its own rate of production.

SUMMARY OF THE CONTROL
OF SODIUM EXCRETION

The control of sodium excretion depends upon the control of two variables of renal function, the GFR and the rate of sodium reabsorption.
The latter is controlled in part by the renin-angiotensin-aldosterone hormone system and, in part, by the factors collectively known as third
factor. In fact, third factor consists of multiple factors, including changes
in intrarenal hydrostatic and oncotic pressures, the distribution of blood
flow within the kidney, and possibly a natriuretic, or salt-losing hormone. The renal sympathetic nerves play a prominent role in each of the
following: the control of aldosterone via renin-angiotensin, the determination of the peritubular Starling pressures within the kidney, and the
control of GFR. Yet, because of the many other known and unknown
factors involved, a transplanted and, therefore, denervated kidney maintains sodium homeostasis quite well.
    The reflexes which control both GFR and sodium reabsorption are
essentially blood-pressure-regulating reflexes, since they are probably
most frequently initiated by changes in arterial or venous pressure or in
cardiac output. This is fitting since cardiovascular function depends
upon an adequate plasma volume, which, as a component of the extracellular-fluid volume, normally reflects the mass of sodium in the
body. In normal persons, these regulatory mechanisms are so precise
that sodium balance does not vary by more than 2 percent despite

marked changes in dietary intake or losses due to sweating, vomiting, diarrhea, hemorrhage, or burns.

In several types of disease, however, sodium balance becomes deranged by the failure of the kidneys to excrete sodium normally. Sodium excretion may fall virtually to zero and remain there despite continued sodium ingestion, and the patient retains large quantities of sodium and water within the body leading to abnormal expansion of extracellular fluid and formation of edema. An important example of this phenomenon is congestive heart failure. A patient with a failing heart (i.e., a heart whose contractility is too low to maintain the cardiac output required for the body's metabolic requirements) usually manifests decreased GFR and increased activity of the renin-angiotensin-aldosterone system, both of which contribute to the virtual absence of sodium from his urine. In addition, his renal filtration fraction is almost always increased—a situation that causes increased oncotic pressure in the peritubular capillaries. The latter and perhaps other sodium-retaining factors contribute to his almost complete reabsorption of sodium. (The net result is expansion of plasma volume, increased capillary pressure, and filtration of fluid into the interstitial space, i.e., edema.)

Why do these sodium-retaining reflexes continue to be elicited despite the fact that the person is in markedly positive and progressively increasing sodium balance? The answer stems from the fact, described earlier, that total extracellular volume, itself, is not directly monitored. In the normal person there is no discrepancy between changes in total extracellular volume and total body sodium, on the one hand, and plasma volume, cardiovascular pressures, and cardiac output, on the other. Thus, a reflex triggered by a change in these latter derivative functions will end up homeostatically regulating body sodium and extracellular volume. In contrast, because of his failing heart, there is a discontinuity between these two groups of variables; e.g., the patient has an inadequate cardiac output despite an increased extracellular volume. In some manner, this reduced cardiac output (or some closely related variable) is detected and initiates sodium-retaining reflexes just as would occur in a normal person whose cardiac output had been reduced due to hemorrhage or severe diarrhea.

There are several other conditions, specifically the liver disease cirrhosis and the kidney disease nephrosis, that tend to produce sodium retention of this kind. They, too, are characterized by persistent sodium-retaining reflexes (decreased GFR, increased aldosterone, etc.). Despite progressive overexpansion of extracellular fluid and formation of edema, as in congestive heart failure, certain receptors must be persistently signaling sodium depletion despite the existence of just the opposite, i.e., positive sodium balance.

All these conditions, including congestive heart failure, are sometimes called diseases of *secondary hyperaldosteronism* because they are usually associated with increased secretion of aldosterone *secondary* to increased renin, which in turn is due to the inappropriate reflexes just described. At one time it was thought that the elevated aldosterone was sufficient in itself to cause progressive accumulation of sodium. It is now recognized that such is not the case and that third factor must also be operating to maintain the retention. This is nicely illustrated by the difference in sodium handling between *primary hyperaldosteronism* and the diseases of secondary hyperaldosteronism. Primary hyperaldosteronism is characterized by persistent oversecretion of aldosterone due to a primary adrenal defect, usually an aldosterone-producing tumor. Because of the increased aldosterone, sodium retention does initially occur, but after a few days, there occurs an *escape* from the effects of aldosterone, i.e., a return to normal sodium excretion despite the continued presence of increased aldosterone. (After balance is reestablished, a persistent, small, positive sodium balance does remain.) What has happened is that the initial sodium retention causes expansion of extracellular volume and total body sodium which then initiates sodium-losing reflexes via changes in GFR and third factor. In other words, persistent, progressive sodium retention cannot be induced by an abnormality in only one of the factors controlling sodium excretion, since reflexes will rapidly be induced whereby opposing changes in the other factors will restore normal sodium excretion. Only when essentially all inputs are altering sodium excretion, either appropriately, as in sodium depletion, or inappropriately, as in the diseases of secondary hyperaldosteronism, will sodium excretion remain continuously near zero.

ADH SECRETION AND EXTRACELLULAR VOLUME

Although we have spoken of extracellular-volume regulation only in terms of the control of sodium excretion, it is clear that, to be most effective in altering extracellular volume, the changes in sodium excretion must be accompanied by equivalent changes in water excretion. We have already pointed out that the ability of water to follow when sodium is reabsorbed depends upon ADH. Accordingly, a decreased extracellular volume must reflexly call forth increased ADH production as well as increased aldosterone secretion. What is the nature of this reflex? ADH is an octapeptide produced by a discrete group of hypothalamic neurons whose cell bodies are located in the supraoptic and paraventricular nuclei and whose axons terminate in the posterior pituitary, from which ADH is released into the blood. These hypothalamic cells receive input from several vascular baroreceptors, particularly a

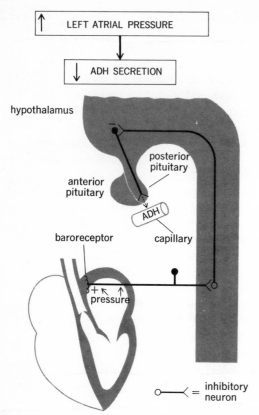

Figure 23   Pathway by which ADH secretion is decreased when plasma volume is increased. The greater plasma volume raises left atrial pressure, which stimulates the atrial baroreceptors and inhibits ADH secretion. (*From A. J. Vander et al., "Human Physiology," © 1970 by McGraw-Hill, Inc. Used with permission of McGraw-Hill Book Company.*)

group located in the left atrium (Fig. 23). The baroreceptors are stimulated by increased atrial blood pressure, and the impulses resulting from this stimulation are transmitted via afferent nerves and ascending pathways to the hypothalamus, where they inhibit the ADH-producing cells. Conversely, decreased atrial pressure causes less firing by the baroreceptors and a resulting stimulation of ADH synthesis and release (Fig. 24). The adaptive value of this baroreceptor reflex should require no comment.[1]

___

[1] Interestingly, angiotensin stimulates ADH release, just as it does aldosterone secretion. Thus, the renin-angiotensin system may play a role in enhancing water reabsorption (via ADH) as it does sodium (via aldosterone). The quantitative significance of this pathway is unclear.

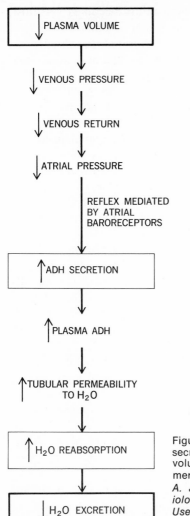

Figure 24 Pathway by which ADH secretion is increased when plasma volume decreases. This figure is merely the converse of Fig. 23. (*From A. J. Vander et al., "Human Physiology," © 1970 by McGraw-Hill, Inc. Used with permission of McGraw-Hill Book Company.*)

ADH AND THE RENAL REGULATION OF EXTRACELLULAR OSMOLARITY

We turn now to the renal compensation for pure-water losses or gains, e.g., the situation in which a man drinks 2 liters of water, but no change in the total salt content of his body occurs. Only his total water changes. The most efficient compensatory mechanism is for the kidneys to excrete the excess water without altering its usual excretion of salt, and this is precisely what they do. ADH secretion is reflexly inhibited, as will be described below, tubular water permeability becomes very low, sodium reabsorption proceeds normally but water is unable to follow, and a large volume of extremely dilute urine is excreted. In this manner, the excess pure water is eliminated. Conversely, when a pure-water deficit occurs, ADH secretion is reflexly stimulated, tubular water permeability is very great, water reabsorption occurs at a maximal rate, the final urine volume becomes extremely small, and its osmolarity is considerably greater than that of the plasma. By this means, relatively less of the filtered water than solute is excreted—which is equivalent to adding pure water to the body—and the pure water deficit is compensated. For example, the excretion of 1 liter of urine having an osmolarity of 1,200 mOsm/liter has the same effect on body-fluid osmolarity as would adding 3 liters of pure water to the body, since a total of 900 mOsm of pure solute have been excreted above and beyond the 300 mOsm of solute required for isoosmolarity of the liter of urine.

To reiterate, pure-water deficits or gains are compensated by partially dissociating water excretion from that of salt through changes in ADH secretion. What receptor input controls ADH under such conditions? The answer is: changes in body-fluid osmolarity. The adaptive rationale should be obvious, since osmolarity is the variable most affected by pure-water gains or deficits. What are the pathways by which osmolarity controls the hypothalamic ADH-producing cells? If osmolarity is the parameter being regulated, it follows that receptors must exist which are sensitive to osmolarity. These osmoreceptors are located in the hypothalamus, but the mechanism by which they detect changes in osmolarity are unknown. The hypothalamic cells which secrete ADH receive neural input from these osmoreceptors. Via these connections an increase in osmolarity stimulates them and increases their rate of ADH secretion; conversely, decreased osmolarity inhibits ADH secretion (Fig. 25).

We have now described two different afferent pathways controlling the ADH-secreting hypothalamic cells, one from baroreceptors and one from osmoreceptors. These hypothalamic cells are therefore true integrating centers whose rate of activity is determined by the total synaptic input. Thus, a simultaneous increase in extracellular volume and decrease in extracellular osmolarity causes maximal inhibition of ADH secretion; conversely, the opposite changes produce maximal stimulation. But what happens in the following situation? A person suffering from severe diarrhea loses 3 liters of salt and water during the same time that he drinks 2 liters of pure water. His total extracellular volume is decreased, but his osmolarity is also decreased. As a result, the ADH-producing cells receive opposing input from the baroreceptors and osmoreceptors. Which predominates depends completely upon the strength of the two inputs.

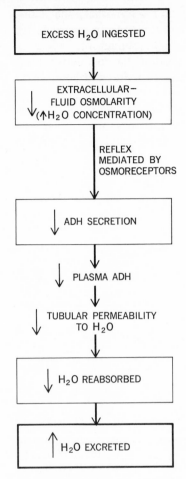

Figure 25 Pathway by which ADH secretion is lowered and water excretion raised when excess water is ingested. (*From A. J. Vander et al., "Human Physiology,"* © *1970 by McGraw-Hill, Inc. Used with permission of McGraw-Hill Book Company.*)

To add to the complexity, these cells receive synaptic input from many other brain areas; thus ADH secretion and, therefore, urine flow can be altered by pain, fear, and a variety of other factors. However, these effects are usually short-lived and should not obscure the generalization that ADH secretion is determined primarily by the states of extracellular volume and osmolarity. Alcohol is a powerful inhibitor of ADH release—a fact that probably accounts for much of the large urine flow accompanying the ingestion of alcohol.

The disease diabetes insipidus, which is different from diabetes mellitus, or sugar diabetes, illustrates what happens when the ADH system is disrupted. Diabetes insipidus is characterized by the constant excretion of a large volume of highly dilute urine (as much as 25 liters/day). In most cases, the flow can be restored to normal by the administration of ADH. These patients apparently have lost the ability to produce ADH, usually as a result of damage to the hypothalamus. Thus, renal tubular permeability to water is low and unchanging regardless of extracellular osmolarity or volume. The very thought of having to urinate (and therefore to drink) 25 liters of water per day underscores the importance of ADH in the control of renal function and body water balance.

Figure 26 shows all those factors known to control renal sodium-and-water excretion in response to severe sweating, as in exercise; the renal retention of fluid helps to compensate for the water and salt lost in the sweat.

THIRST AND SALT APPETITE

Now we must turn to the other component of the balance — control of intake. It should be evident that large deficits of salt and water can be only partly compensated by renal conservation and that ingestion is the ultimate compensatory mechanism. The subjective feeling of thirst, which drives one to obtain and ingest water, is stimulated both by a reduced extracellular volume and by an increased plasma osmolarity. The adaptive significance of both are self-evident. Note that these are precisely the same changes which stimulate ADH production. The centers which mediate thirst are located in the hypothalamus and are very close to those areas which produce ADH. They are also very close to, but distinct from, food-intake centers. Damage to the thirst centers abolishes water intake completely. Conversely, electric stimulation of them may induce profound and prolonged drinking.

Because of the similarities between the stimuli for ADH secretion and for thirst, it is tempting to speculate that the receptors (osmoreceptors and atrial baroreceptors) which initiate the ADH-controlling reflexes are identical to those for thirst. This may, indeed, be the case, but there are also other pathways controlling thirst. For example, dryness of the mouth and throat causes profound thirst, which is relieved by merely moistening them. It is fascinating that, when animals such as the camel (and man, to a lesser extent) become markedly dehydrated, they will rapidly drink just enough water to replace their previous losses and then stop. What is amazing is that, when they stop, the water has not yet had time to be absorbed from the gastrointestinal tract into the blood. Some kind of metering of the water intake by the gastrointestinal tract has occurred, but its nature remains a mystery.

Figure 26   Pathways by which sodium and water excretion are decreased in response to severe sweating. This figure is an amalgamation of Figs. 17, 18, 19, and 20 and the converse of Fig. 25. The possible contribution of a natriuretic hormone and of as yet unidentified humoral vasoactive agents are not shown. (*Modified from A. J. Vander et al., "Human Physiology,"* © *1970 by McGraw-Hill, Inc. Used with permission of McGraw-Hill Book Company.*)

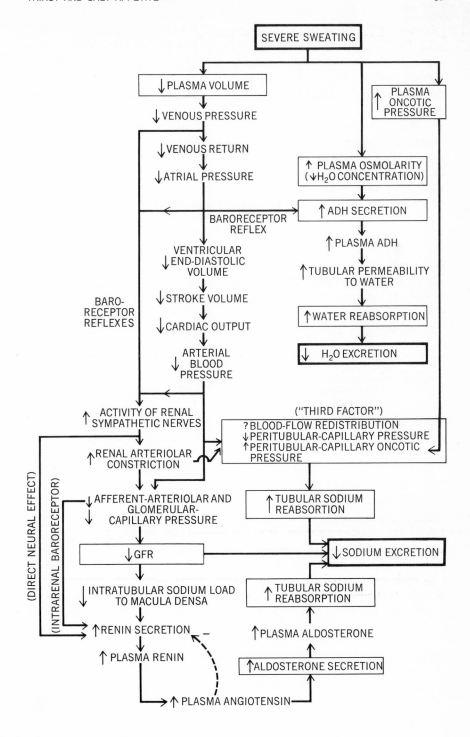

A recent finding of considerable interest is that angiotensin stimulates both thirst and ADH secretion by a direct effect on the brain. Thus, the renin-angiotensin system is an important regulator not only of sodium balance but of water balance as well and constitutes one of the pathways by which thirst and ADH secretion are stimulated when extracellular volume is decreased.

Salt appetite, which is the analogue of thirst, is also an extremely important component of sodium homeostasis in most mammals, particularly in the herbivores. It is clear that salt appetite is innate and consists of two components: hedonistic appetite and regulatory appetite. In other words, animals like salt and eat it whenever they can, regardless of whether they are salt-deficient, and, in addition, their drive to obtain salt is markedly increased in the presence of deficiency. The significance of these animal studies for man is unclear. Salt craving does seem to occur in humans who are severely salt-depleted, but the contribution of regulatory salt appetite to everyday sodium homeostasis in normal persons is probably slight. On the other hand, man does seem to have a strong hedonistic appetite for salt, as manifested by almost universally large intakes of sodium whenever it is cheap and readily available. Thus, the average American intake of salt is 10 to 15 gm/day despite the fact that humans can survive quite normally on less than 0.5 gm/day. Present evidence strongly suggests that a large salt intake may be an important contributor to the pathogenesis of hypertension.

Study questions: **22** to **35**

Chapter 7

Renal Regulation
of Potassium Balance

OBJECTIVES

The student understands the renal regulation of potassium.
1   Describes the basic renal processes for handling potassium
2   Contrasts the contribution of each nephron site to potassium handling
    during a high and low potassium diet
3   Describes the mechanism by which potassium secretion is accomplished
    by the distal tubule
4   Lists the inputs which control the rate of potassium secretion by the
    distal tubule
5   Describes the pathway by which changes in potassium balance influence
    aldosterone secretion
6   Describes the effects of alkalosis on potassium secretion and balance
7   Describes the relationship between renal sodium handling and potas-
    sium secretion
8   Describes the effects of unreabsorbed anions on potassium secretion
    and balance
9   Predicts the changes in potassium secretion and balance occurring in
    representative abnormal situations: respiratory or metabolic alkalosis,
    primary aldosteronism, diarrhea, diabetes mellitus

The potassium concentration of the extracellular fluid is a closely regulated quantity. The importance of maintaining this concentration in the internal environment stems primarily from the role of potassium in the excitability of nerve and muscle. The resting membrane potentials of these tissues are directly related to the ratio of intracellular-to-extracellular potassium concentration. Raising the external potassium concentration lowers the resting membrane potential, thus increasing cell excitability. Conversely, lowering the external potassium hyperpolarizes cell membranes and reduces their excitability.

Since most of the body's potassium is found within cells, primarily as a result of active-ion-transport systems located in cell membranes, even a slight alteration of rates of ion transport across cell membranes can produce a large change in the amount of extracellular potassium. Unfortunately, relatively little is known about the physiological control of these transport mechanisms, and, obviously, our understanding of the regulation of extracellular potassium concentration will remain incomplete until further data are obtained on this critical subject.

The normal person remains in potassium balance (as he does in sodium balance) by excreting daily an amount of potassium equal to the amount of potassium ingested minus the small amounts eliminated in the feces and sweat. Normally potassium losses via sweat and the gastrointestinal tract are small, although large quantities can be lost by the latter during vomiting or diarrhea. Again, the control of renal function is the major mechanism by which body potassium is regulated.

Potassium is completely filterable at the glomerulus. The amounts of potassium excreted in the urine are generally a small fraction (10 to 15 percent) of the filtered quantity. These facts establish the existence of tubular potassium reabsorption. However, it has also been demonstrated that under certain conditions the excreted quantity may actually exceed the filtered quantity. We therefore conclude that tubular potassium secretion also exists. Thus the subject is complicated by the fact that potassium can be both reabsorbed and secreted by the tubule.

The tubular reabsorption of potassium is accomplished by active transport, which occurs in all nephron segments except the descending loop of Henle. The quantitative contributions of the various nephron segments to reabsorption are quite similar to those for sodium. Approximately 65 percent of the total filtered potassium is reabsorbed by the proximal tubule and another 20 to 30 percent by the ascending loop of Henle. Thus, only about 10 percent of the filtered potassium enters the distal tubule. Present evidence indicates that the reabsorption of this 90 percent of the filtered potassium by the proximal tubule and loop occurs at virtually the same rate regardless of changes in body potassium. In other words the reabsorption of potassium by these nephron segments does not seem to be controlled so as to achieve potassium homeostasis.

The situation for the distal tubule and collecting ducts is quite different. First, they are able both to secrete and to reabsorb potassium. Moreover, the rate at which at least one of these opposing processes (secretion) occurs is variable; accordingly, the *net* contribution of these nephron segments may be either reabsorption or secretion. It is by alteration of this mix in the distal tubule (and to a lesser extent in the collecting duct) that changes in potassium excretion are achieved.

Let us take a few examples. During potassium deprivation (caused, for example, by a low-potassium diet), the homeostatic response is to reduce potassium excretion to a minimal level. Using micropuncture to evaluate potassium handling by each nephron segment, we would find that the proximal tubule and loop were reabsorbing about 90 percent of the filtered potassium and that the distal tuble and collecting duct were reabsorbing most of the remaining 10 percent, so that very little potassium was excreted. Now we shift to the opposite end of the spectrum and look at the kidneys during a high-potassium diet. In this case the homeostatic response is to excrete large quantities of potassium so as to balance output with intake. Micropuncture reveals that the proximal tubule and the loop are still reabsorbing the same fraction (90 percent) of filtered potassium so that the amount of potassium entering the distal tubule from the loop is not much different from the amount entering it when the individual was on the low-potassium diet. Now the radical difference appears: The distal tubule manifests net secretion of potassium rather than the net reabsorption seen on the low-potassium diet. Indeed the quantity of potassium added to the distal lumen by secretion may be greater than the quantity of potassium reabsorbed upstream by the proximal tubule and loop—the result being *net secretion* by the overall nephron, i.e., the *excretion* of more potassium, than was *filtered.*[1]

These examples should reinforce the fact that normally the control of renal potassium excretion resides in the distal portions of the nephron, particularly in the distal tubule, whose contribution can be either net reabsorption or secretion. It seems likely that the major controlled variable is the rate of secretion; i.e., that the rate of reabsorption in this segment, as in the proximal tubule and loop, occurs at a relatively fixed rate despite changes in physiological conditions and that superimposed upon it is a variable degree of tubular secretion. Depending upon the rate of secretion, the net distal contribution can be reabsorption, no change, or secretion. A very useful simplifying assumption emerges: In describing the homeostatic control of potassium excretion we may ignore changes in GFR or in reabsorption and focus only on the factors

---

[1] The collecting duct handles potassium in much the same way that the distal tubule does. However, there seem to be certain interesting differences. The distal tubule is quantitatively the more important, and we have chosen to focus on it. (See Stein and Reineck, 1974, in Suggested Readings for Chap. 7.)

which alter the rate of distal potassium secretion. It must be pointed out, however, that under certain abnormal conditions potassium reabsorption in the proximal tubule or loop may be decreased and that a large quantity of the potassium excreted may represent filtered potassium which is not reabsorbed. One such situation is osmotic diuresis. Just as was true for sodium, the presence of an osmotic diuretic interferes with potassium reabsorption; this is one reason for the marked urinary loss of potassium suffered by patients with uncontrolled diabetes mellitus.

POTASSIUM SECRETION

To reiterate, potassium secretion can occur in the distal tubules and, to a lesser extent, in the collecting ducts. The process by which potassium secretion occurs is still controversial but, at least in the distal tubule, probably involves active transport of potassium across the peritubular cell membrane (i.e., the membrane separating cell from interstitial fluid) and into the distal-tubule cell followed by passive diffusion out of the cell and into the lumen. The passive step is driven by the high concentration gradient from cell to lumen achieved by the peritubular-membrane pump. In addition, recall that there exists an electric potential difference between the distal-tubule (or collecting-duct) lumen and the interstitial fluid of approximately -50 mV, the lumen being negative. This PD acts as a second driving force for passive potassium entry.[1]

Given this model, one can perceive the major factors which directly determine the rate of potassium secretion: (1) the potassium concentration gradient between the interior of the cell and the lumen, which determines the concentration force for passive entry into the lumen; (2) the tubular potential difference, which determines the electric force for passive entry and; (3) the permeability of the luminal membrane to potassium. In the next section we describe the various situations in which the rate of potassium secretion is altered. In each case, one or more of the three factors described above must constitute the mechanism by which the altered secretion is mediated, although frequently we are not yet certain as to the relative importance of each in any given situation.

HOMEOSTATIC CONTROL OF SECRETION

What are the factors which influence secretion so as to achieve homeostasis of body potassium? In other words, how do changes in body potassium induce the kidney to secrete more or less potassium? One of

[1] For a rigorous analysis of potassium movements and the PDs in the distal tubule, see Brenner and Berliner, 1973, and Giebisch, 1971, in Suggested Readings for Chap. 7.

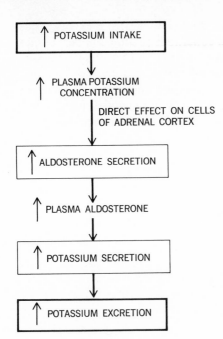

Figure 27 Aldosterone-mediated pathway by which an increased potassium intake induces greater potassium excretion. (*From A. J. Vander et al., "Human Physiology,"* © *1970 by McGraw Hill, Inc. Used with permission of McGraw-Hill Book Company.*)

the most important links is via direct changes in the potassium concentration of the distal-tubular cells. For example, when a high potassium diet is ingested, potassium concentration in most of the body's cells increases, including the renal tubular cells. This higher concentration enhances the gradient for potassium secretion into the lumen and raises potassium excretion. Conversely, a low-potassium diet or a negative potassium balance, e.g., from diarrhea, lowers renal-tubular-cell potassium concentration; this reduces potassium secretion and excretion, thereby helping to reestablish potassium balance.

A second important factor linking potassium secretion to potassium balance is the hormone aldosterone, which, besides stimulating tubular sodium reabsorption, simultaneously enhances tubular potassium secretion. The reflex by which changes in extracellular volume control aldosterone production is completely different from the reflex initiated by an excess or deficit of potassium. The former constitutes a complex pathway, involving renin and angiotensin. The latter, however, seems to be much simpler and works in the following way (Fig. 27): The aldosterone-secreting cells of the adrenal cortex are apparently sensitive to the potassium concentration of the extracellular fluid bathing them. Or, more likely, they are sensitive to their own intracellular potassium concentration. Thus, an increased intake of potassium leads to an increased extracellular potassium concentration, which in turn directly stimulates aldosterone production by the adrenal cortex. This extra aldosterone circulates to the kidney, where it increases potassium secretion by the distal portions of the nephron and thereby eliminates the excess potassium from the body. Aldosterone may act by stimulating the peritubular-membrane potassium pump; such would increase intracellular potassium concentration and the gradient for movement into the lumen. Conversely, a lowered extracellular potassium concentration decreases aldosterone production and thereby inhibits tubular potassium secretion. Less potassium than usual is excreted in the urine, thus helping to restore

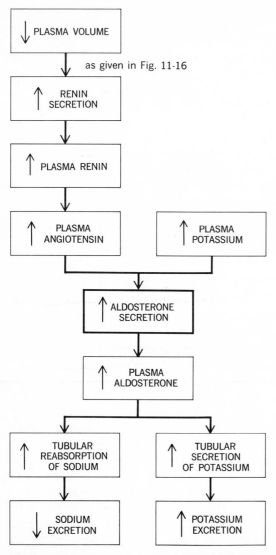

Figure 28 Summary of the control of aldosterone and its functions. (*From A. J. Vander et al., "Human Physiology," © 1970 by McGraw-Hill, Inc. Used with permission of McGraw-Hill Book Company.*)

the normal extracellular potassium concentration. Complete restoration of body potassium depends upon the ingestion of additional potassium.

The control and renal tubular effects of aldosterone are summarized in Figure 28. It should be evident that a conflict will arise if increases in potassium and extracellular volume occur simultaneously, since these two changes drive aldosterone production in opposite directions. The adaptive value, if any, of such a potential conflict is at present unknown. We mention the problem primarily as a reminder that different homeostatic mechanisms frequently conflict with each other and that the ability of any living organism to survive ultimately depends upon whether it can resolve such conflicts by integrating the opposing demands.

We have now described the mechanisms by which potassium secretion is controlled so as to achieve potassium homeostasis. However, the fact is that potassium secretion is also influenced by factors *not* designed to maintain body potassium constant, namely, by extracellular-volume changes, acid-base disturbances, the presence of poorly reabsorbed anions, and diuretic drugs. In particular, we shall see that, because the renal mechanisms for potassium are intimately related to those for sodium and hydrogen ion, potassium balance can frequently be upset as a result of the homeostatic mechanisms regulating these other ions. The aldosterone conflict described above is one example, but there are others of greater importance.

OTHER FACTORS INFLUENCING POTASSIUM SECRETION

Acid-Base Changes

The empirical finding is as follows: The existence of an alkalosis, either metabolic or respiratory in origin, induces increased potassium secretion and excretion. (The opposite is true for certain kinds of acidosis, especially when they are acute. However, the analysis of potassium excretion in acidosis is quite complicated and no simple generalization is very useful.) Thus, a primary disturbance in a person's acid-base status can result in a secondary disturbance in his potassium balance. For example, a patient suffering from metabolic alkalosis (induced, say, by vomiting) will manifest increased urinary excretion of potassium solely as a result of the alkalosis and will, therefore, become potassium deficient. Of course, as soon as potassium balance is upset by these events, the mechanisms described above (renal-cell potassium concentration and aldosterone secretion) will be triggered so as to limit the imbalance.

The effects of acid-base disturbances on potassium secretion appear to be mediated, at least in part, through changes in the potassium concentration of distal-tubular cells. Present evidence indicates that the presence of a renal intracellular alkalosis somehow causes an increase in cell potassium concentration and, thereby, its rate of secretion. (Perhaps renal intracellular alkalosis stimulates the peritubular potassium pump.)

Finally, it should be emphasized that this relationship is only one side of the coin; we shall describe later how primary changes in potassium balance induce secondary changes in the renal handling of hydrogen ion.

Renal Sodium Handling

A common denominator of many observations is that potassium secretion is usually elevated in the presence of a high rate of sodium excretion. For example, the administration of diuretics (drugs which directly block sodium reabsorption) frequently causes a marked increase in the excretion of potassium as well as of sodium. Conversely, when the urine is virtually sodium-free (as, for example, in marked salt depletion), potassium secretion may be reduced—a phenomenon which can lead to potassium retention. This last fact is particularly puzzling, since salt depletion induces increased secretion of aldosterone, which should then stimulate potassium secretion. In spite of this, potassium secretion may remain relatively low.

The mechanisms responsible for the correspondence between sodium and distal-tubular potassium secretion are multiple and still unclear. One critical factor may well be the volume of fluid flow through the distal tubule. At least this factor has good predictive value, for the volume of fluid flow is increased by osmotic diuretics, diuretic drugs, a high-salt diet, and the escape phase of primary hyperaldosteronism—all situations in which potassium secretion is enhanced. Conversely the volume of distal-tubular fluid flow is decreased on a low-sodium diet and in secondary hyperaldosteronism with edema—both situations in which potassium secretion and excretion are relatively normal despite the increased aldosterone and may actually be subnormal so as to cause some degree of potassium retention.

That the volume of fluid flow through the distal tubule might influence potassium secretion may be explained by the fact that, as mentioned above, potassium entry into the lumen from the cell is a passive process. Accordingly, a large fluid volume would keep the intraluminal potassium concentration low and thereby enhance the gradient for passive potassium entry. A low volume of fluid flow would have just the opposite effect.[1]

Unreabsorbed Anions

Another factor which can effectively increase potassium secretion and excretion is the presence within the distal tubule of large quantities of

[1] The relationship between the renal handling of sodium chloride and potassium is not a one-way street. We have described the effects of changes in salt balance and in tubular flow rates on potassium secretion because of their clear-cut clinical significance. However, it is also true that primary changes in potassium balance may have important effects on sodium reabsorption by multiple mechanisms. The text describes one of the indirect influences resulting from potassium-induced changes in aldosterone. There are others, including direct effects of potassium both on tubular sodium reabsorption and on renin secretion. (See Laragh and Sealey, 1973, in Suggested Readings for Chap. 6.)

unreabsorbed anions. The most important situation in which this occurs is diabetic ketoacidosis, in which keto acid anions are filtered in such large quantities that the tubular transport maximum for them is exceeded and large quantities remain as the fluid flows through the distal tubule. Their presence causes increased amounts of potassium to move into the lumen (secretion) and to be excreted. (This *increased secretion* is a second cause of potassium depletion in uncontrolled diabetes. The first cause is *reduced reabsorption* of potassium secondary to the osmotic-diuretic effect of the unreabsorbed glucose and keto acids.)

The ability of large quantities of unreabsorbed anions to enhance potassium secretion is best explained by their effect on the tubular PD. As active sodium transport continues in the distal tubule, the inability of these anions to follow the sodium causes the lumen of the tubule to become more negatively charged; this increased negativity acts as a force to drive potassium into the lumen.

Effects of Diuretic Drugs

As described earlier, diuretic drugs are frequently used clinically to inhibit tubular sodium reabsorption. These drugs almost invariably also influence potassium secretion (and, thereby, excretion), and a brief discussion of their effects may help to emphasize the major factors which influence potassium secretion.

On first thought, one might predict that all diuretic drugs would enhance potassium secretion, since by inhibiting sodium and, therefore, water reabsorption, they all enhance fluid flow through the distal tubule. The observed fact is that many do, but others actually inhibit potassium secretion. Clearly, then, these latter drugs must exert an additional effect on potassium secretion that is strong enough to more than offset the secretion-enhancing effect of the increased fluid flow. Spironolactone is a diuretic which inhibits the action of aldosterone on the renal tubule; accordingly it also inhibits potassium secretion by blocking aldosterone's stimulatory effect. Mercurial diuretics inhibit the peritubular membrane pump for potassium and thereby decrease cell potassium concentration and the gradient for diffusion into the lumen. Amiloride, another diuretic, in some unknown manner reduces the luminal negativity and therefore reduces the electric gradient for entry into the lumen.

Finally, certain diuretics increase potassium secretion much *more* than would be expected by the fluid-flow effect alone. These agents are inhibitors of the enzyme carbonic anhydrase, and, for reasons to be described in the next section, they increase intracellular potassium concentration, thereby increasing the gradient for entry into the lumen.

Study questions: **36** to **39**

ALDACTAZide > spironolactone
AldacTone

Chapter 8

Renal Regulation of Extracellular Hydrogen-ion Concentration

OBJECTIVES

The student understands the renal regulation of extracellular pH.
1 States the role of the kidneys in the regulation of extracellular pH
2 States the two ways in which the kidneys perform this role
3 Calculates the mass of bicarbonate filtered each day
4 Describes the acidifying effect of renal bicarbonate loss
5 Describes the mechanism by which tubular bicarbonate reabsorption occurs; states the role of carbonic anhydrase
6 Describes how tubular acid secretion can add new bicarbonate to the blood, i.e., lead to the excretion of hydrogen ion
7 States the limiting urine pH, the reason for it, and its significance
8 Defines titratable acid and describes how the measurement is made; states the major buffer(s) which contributes to the formation of titratable acid and its quantitative contributions
9 Describes the role of ammonia in the contribution of new bicarbonate to the blood; defines diffusion trapping and describes how it explains the relationship between urine pH and ammonium excretion; defines ammonia adaptation to chronic acidosis

10 Distinguishes the rates of acid secretion and excretion

11 Calculates, given data, the rate of total acid secretion

12 Calculates, given data, the rate at which the kidneys contribute new bicarbonate to the blood (acid excretion)

13 Describes glomerulotubular balance for bicarbonate

14 Describes the relationship between blood Pco_2 and tubular acid secretion

15 Lists the changes (increase or decrease) of acid secretion, titratable acid excretion, bicarbonate excretion, ammonium excretion, renal addition of new bicarbonate to the blood, and plasma bicarbonate in: metabolic acidosis, metabolic alkalosis, respiratory acidosis, respiratory alkalosis

16 Describes the influence of extracellular-volume contraction on acid secretion and the capacity of the kidneys to repair an alkalosis

17 Describes the influence of potassium balance on acid secretion and the resulting effect on acid-base balance

18 Describes how primary changes in acid secretion can influence sodium and chloride reabsorption

19 Describes the urine findings in a patient treated with a carbonic anhydrase inhibitor and the mechanisms responsible

The homeostatic control of hydrogen-ion concentration in the body fluids is accomplished primarily by regulation of the carbon dioxide–bicarbonate buffer system:

$$H_2O + CO_2 \rightleftharpoons H_2CO_3 \rightleftharpoons H^+ + HCO_3^-$$

There are, of course, other buffer systems in the body, but they are all in equilibrium with each other; therefore, a change in one buffer pair causes parallel changes in the other buffer systems. In other words, the hydrogen-ion concentration can be fixed by manipulating the concentrations of the components of a single buffer system. There are extremely precise physiological mechanisms for regulating the carbon dioxide–bicarbonate system; the Pco_2 is regulated by the respiratory system, and the bicarbonate concentration by the kidneys.

The kidneys perform their function in two major ways: (1) variable reabsorption of the bicarbonate filtered at the glomerulus, and (2) addition of *new* bicarbonate to the plasma flowing through the kidneys. As we shall see, these two processes are totally interrelated and are, in fact, accomplished by a single mechanism. Inspection of the carbon dioxide–bicarbonate equation above makes it obvious how control of these two renal processes homeostatically regulates extracellular-fluid hydrogen-ion concentration. When plasma hydrogen-ion concentration has been reduced (alkalosis), it can be raised back toward normal by lowering plasma bicarbonate concentration, thereby driving the reaction to the right and generating more hydrogen ion; this the kidneys do by failing to reabsorb all the filtered bicarbonate during alkalosis, allowing this unreabsorbed bicarbonate to be excreted in the urine. *In essence, the excretion of a bicarbonate ion in the urine has virtually the same effect on the blood as would adding a hydrogen ion to the blood.* In contrast to this renal compensation for alkalosis, when plasma hydrogen-ion concentration has been increased (acidosis), the kidneys reabsorb all the filtered bicarbonate and, in addition, contribute new bicarbonate ions (produced by the renal tubular cells) to the blood, thereby shifting the reaction to the left and returning plasma pH toward normal. As we shall see, the renal addition of new bicarbonate to the blood is associated with the excretion of an equal amount of acid in the urine; "the kidney has added new bicarbonate to the blood" and "the kidney has *excreted acid*" are synonymous statements. (Throughout this section the reader must be careful to distinguish between "secretion" and "excretion." Thus, to compensate for acidosis, the kidneys excrete an acid urine and alkalinize the blood; in response to alkalosis, they excrete an alkaline urine and acidify the blood.)

BICARBONATE REABSORPTION

Bicarbonate is completely filterable at the glomerulus. How much is normally filtered per day?

$$\text{Filtered } HCO_3^-/\text{day} = GFR \times P_{HCO_3^-}$$
$$= 180 \text{ liters/day} \times 24 \text{ mEq/liter}$$
$$= 4{,}320 \text{ mEq/day}$$

Zero reabsorption of this bicarbonate would be tantamount to adding more than 4 liters of $1 \, N$ acid to the body. In a normal person, i.e., in the absence of alkalosis, virtually all is reabsorbed. Thus, the reabsorption of bicarbonate is normally a conservation process, and essentially none appears in the urine.

How is bicarbonate reabsorbed? One might naturally assume that reabsorption of bicarbonate occurs passively as a result of the same forces described earlier for chloride. Such is not the case,[1] however. Passive reabsorption requires that the tubule be quite permeable to the ion in question. The tubule is quite permeable to the chloride ion, but it is relatively impermeable to the bicarbonate ion. Accordingly, the reabsorption of bicarbonate is an active process, but it is not accomplished in the conventional manner of simply having an active pump for bicar-

[1] It is probable that a very small fraction of bicarbonate is reabsorbed passively, but this moiety is of negligible significance. (See Rector, 1973, in Suggested Readings for Chap. 8.)

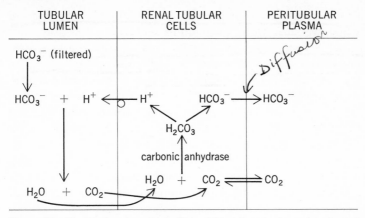

Figure 29   Mechanism by which filtered bicarbonate is reabsorbed. In the scheme illustrated here, H^+ is generated directly by the dissociation of H_2CO_3. In reality the following scheme is more likely: The secreted H^+ is generated from water, and the resulting OH^- is left behind in the cell, where it reacts with the H^+ generated by H_2CO_3 to regenerate water. In either case, the overall effect is, in most respects, the same, so we have used the simpler scheme.

bonate ions. Rather, the mechanism by which bicarbonate is reabsorbed involves hydrogen-ion secretion and is shown in Fig. 29. In studying this complicated figure, begin with the carbon dioxide entering the cell from the peritubular plasma and proceed upwards.

The key elements in this scheme are the intracellular hydration of carbon dioxide (catalyzed by the enzyme, carbonic anhydrase) to carbonic acid, dissociation of the acid to generate hydrogen ion, and the active secretion of this hydrogen ion into the lumen. The bicarbonate generated simultaneously in the cell is transported into the peritubular plasma, probably by diffusion. Once in the tubular lumen, the hydrogen ion combines with a filtered bicarbonate to form carbonic acid; this decomposes to water and carbon dioxide, which diffuse into the cell and then either diffuse into the peritubular plasma or are used by the cell to generate another hydrogen ion. It may seem inaccurate to refer to this process as bicarbonate reabsorption, since the bicarbonate which appears in the peritubular plasma is not the same bicarbonate ion which was filtered. Yet, the overall result is, in effect, the same as it would be if the filtered bicarbonate had been more conventionally reabsorbed like a sodium or potassium ion.

It is also important to note that the hydrogen ion which was *secreted* into the lumen is *not excreted* in the urine. It has been incorporated into water and reabsorbed. The key point here is that any secreted acid (hydrogen ion) which combines with bicarbonate in the lumen to effect bicarbonate reabsorption does not contribute to the urinary *excretion* of acid. Finally, it should be mentioned that the process of acid secretion is intimately related to sodium reabsorption, a problem to which we shall return later in this section.

This process of hydrogen-ion secretion and bicarbonate reabsorption occurs throughout the nephron with the exception of the descending loop of Henle. Quantitatively, the proximal tubule is most important in that it reabsorbs approximately 80 to 90 percent of the filtered bicarbonate. The remaining bicarbonate is normally reabsorbed by the loop of Henle and distal tubule. Throughout the tubule, as shown in the figure, intracellular carbonic anhydrase is involved in the reactions generating hydrogen ion and bicarbonate. In the proximal tubule, carbonic anhydrase is also located in the luminal cell membranes, and this carbonic anhydrase catalyzes the intraluminal decomposition of the very large quantities of carbonic acid formed in this nephron segment.

ADDITION OF NEW BICARBONATE TO THE PLASMA (RENAL EXCRETION OF ACID)

Besides being able to conserve all the filtered bicarbonate, the kidneys can also contribute *new* bicarbonate to the plasma, so that the mass of bicarbonate in the renal veins exceeds that which entered the kidneys originally. The effect of adding new base to the body is, of course, to alkalinize it, and this is the renal compensation for acidosis.

The mechanism by which new bicarbonate is added to the blood is fundamentally the same as that for bicarbonate reabsorption, namely, tubular acid secretion (Fig. 30). The only difference between these two

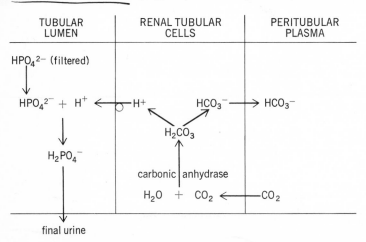

Figure 30 Reaction of secreted hydrogen ion with filtered phosphate. Note that a carbon dioxide has been used up, and a new bicarbonate has been released into the blood. In contrast, Fig. 29 shows that no net gain or loss of carbon dioxide or bicarbonate occurs when the secreted hydrogen ion is used for bicarbonate reabsorption.

processes is a function of the fate of the secreted hydrogen ions within the tubular lumen. In the case of bicarbonate reabsorption, the secreted acid combines with filtered bicarbonate and is reabsorbed as water; whereas, in the case of new-bicarbonate addition to the blood, the secreted acid combines with other buffers in the lumen or, to a very small degree, remains free in solution and is excreted. Let us first consider the case in which the secreted acid combines with phosphate, one of the two most important urinary buffers, the other being ammonia.

Note that the process of hydrogen-ion secretion is the same tubular mechanism described previously, but the net overall effect is different simply because the secreted acid reacts with filtered phosphate rather than with filtered bicarbonate. Therefore, the bicarbonate generated within the tubular cell and entering the plasma constitutes a net gain of bicarbonate by the blood, not merely a replacement for a filtered bicarbonate. Thus, when a secreted hydrogen ion combines in the lumen with a buffer other than bicarbonate, the overall effect is not merely one of bicarbonate conservation but rather of addition to the body of *new* bicarbonate, which raises the bicarbonate concentration of the blood and alkalinizes it.

The figure also demonstrates another important point; namely that the renal contribution of new bicarbonate to the blood is accompanied by the *excretion* of an equivalent amount of acid in the urine. In this case, in contrast to the reabsorption of bicarbonate, the *secreted* hydrogen ion remains in the tubular fluid, trapped there by the phosphate buffer, and is *excreted* in the urine. This should reinforce the concept that, when they add new bicarbonate to the blood, the kidneys are really excreting acid from the body, thereby alkalinizing it.

Figure 31 illustrates the same process but with ammonia rather than phosphate as the intraluminal buffer. Unlike phosphate, ammonia gains entry to the tubular lumen not by filtration but rather by tubular synthesis and secretion, the mechanism of which will be described later. Again we see that the overall effect is the addition of a new bicarbonate to the plasma, combination of the secreted acid with an intralumenal buffer, in this case ammonia, and excretion of the acid.

The type and quantity of buffers is a crucial determinant of the maximal rate at which the kidneys can contribute new bicarbonate to the blood. This stems from the fact that there exists a limiting hydrogen-ion concentration gradient against which net secretion of acid into the lumen can occur. As hydrogen ions are secreted into the lumen, most are removed from solution by combination with the buffers within the tubular fluid, but a very small number remains free in solution so that the pH of the tubular fluid decreases. The minimal pH of human urine is approximately 4.4. At this pH, the *free* hydrogen-ion concentration is 1,000 times greater in the tubular lumen than in the peritubular plasma

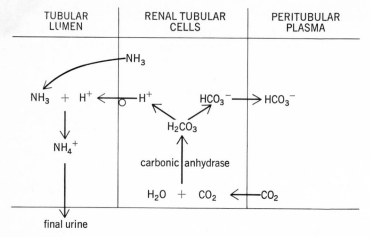

Figure 31   Reaction of secreted hydrogen ion with ammonia formed by tubular cells.

(pH 4.4 versus pH 7.4). This huge concentration gradient causes net passive back-diffusion of hydrogen ion out of the lumen and into the blood at a rate identical to that of active secretion into the lumen. The net result is that the entire process of acid secretion and new-bicarbonate formation is counteracted. The nature and quantity of urinary buffers available to react with the secreted acid and prevent this limiting gradient for free hydrogen ion from being reached is, therefore, of key importance.

Phosphate as a Buffer

The relationship between monobasic and dibasic phosphate is as follows:

$$HPO_4^{2-} + H^+ \rightleftharpoons H_2PO_4^-$$

This buffer pair provides an excellent buffer system because its pK is 6.8. Expressed in Henderson-Hasselbach terms:

$$pH = 6.8 + \log \frac{[HPO_4^{2-}]}{[H_2PO_4^-]}$$

At the normal pH of plasma and, therefore, of the glomerular filtrate, the equation becomes

$$7.4 = 6.8 + \log \frac{[HPO_4^{2-}]}{[H_2PO_4^-]}$$

Solving the equation, we find that there is four times more dibasic (HPO_4^{2-}) than monobasic ($H_2PO_4^-$) phosphate in plasma. Therefore the HPO_4^{2-} is available for buffering secreted hydrogen ions. By the time the minimal pH of 4.4 is reached, virtually all the HPO_4^{2-} has been converted to $H_2PO_4^-$.

How much HPO_4^{2-} is normally filtered per day?

$$\text{Filtered total phosphate/day} = 180 \text{ liters/day} \times 1 \text{ mmol/liter}$$
$$= 180 \text{ mmol/day}$$
$$\text{Filtered } HPO_4^{2-} = 80\% \times 180 \text{ mmol/day}$$
$$= 144 \text{ mmol/day}$$

However, not all of this filtered HPO_4^{2-} is available for buffering, because about 75 percent of filtered phosphate is reabsorbed. Accordingly, unreabsorbed HPO_4^{2-} available for buffering is 0.25×144 mmol/day = 36 mmol/day. Thus, the reabsorption of phosphate considerably limits the supply of HPO_4^{2-} for buffering. Accordingly, as we shall see, ammonia must usually bear the major burden of accepting the additional hydrogen ions in acidosis.

Ammonia and phosphate are normally the only important urinary buffers. However, under abnormal conditions, certain organic buffers may appear in the tubular fluid in large enough quantity to allow them also to act as important buffers. A particularly interesting example is the patient with uncontrolled diabetes mellitus. As a result of insulin deficiency, such a patient may become extremely acidotic because he produces large quantities of the keto acids, acetoacetic and β-hydroxybutyric acid, which, at plasma pH, almost completely dissociate to yield anions (β-hydroxybutyrate and acetoacetate) and hydrogen ions. These anions are filtered at the glomerulus but are only partly reabsorbed, because they are present in great enough quantities to exceed the renal reabsorptive T_m's for them. Accordingly, they are available in the tubular fluid to buffer a portion of the acid being secreted by the tubules to compensate for the acidosis. However, their usefulness in this role is limited by the fact that their pK's are low — approximately 4.5. This means that only half of these anions will be titrated by secreted acid before the limiting urine pH of 4.4 is reached; i.e., only half of them can actually be used as buffers. If the kidneys could lower the luminal pH to 1 as the stomach can, then it could titrate all of the β-hydroxybutyrate.

Ammonia as a Buffer

The ammonia-ammonium reaction has a very high pK, approximately 9.2:

$$NH_3 + H^+ \rightleftharpoons NH_4^+$$

$$pH = 9.2 + \log \frac{[NH_3]}{[NH_4^+]}$$

This means that, given the usual urine pH of 7.4 or less, virtually all NH_3 that gains entry to the tubular lumen will immediately pick up hydrogen ions to form NH_4^+. Accordingly, as long as a supply of NH_3 is available, hydrogen-ion secretion and net addition of bicarbonate to the blood can continue with no danger of reaching the minimal urinary pH.

**Ammonia Synthesis and
Diffusion Trapping**

The source of ammonia is the renal tubular cells, themselves, which form ammonia from glutamine and other amino acids. The major reaction — conversion of glutamine to glutamic acid and ammonia — is catalyzed by the enzyme *glutaminase*. When an individual is acidotic for more than a few days, there occurs a marked increase in ammonia synthesis. This phenomenon, known as *adaptation of ammonia synthesis,* is due, in part, to increased activity of glutaminase, but the mechanism responsible for the increase is unknown. The result of this adaptation is that the increased ammonia synthesis provides more ammonia to act as intraluminal buffer so that the kidneys can compensate for the chronic acidosis by contributing a larger amount of new bicarbonate to the blood.

The mechanism by which ammonia, once having been synthesized within the cell, gains entry to the lumen is of considerable importance (Fig. 32). It is known as *nonionic diffusion,* or *diffusion trapping.* The

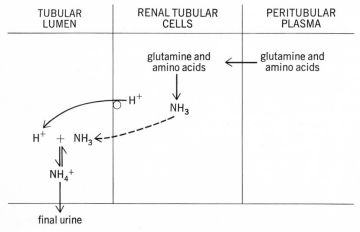

Figure 32   Ammonia synthesis and entry into the tubule.

underlying principles are simple: (1) The ability of a substance to passively penetrate any cell membrane depends upon the lipid solubility of the substance. (2) Ammonia, being nonionized, is highly lipid-soluble; whereas ammonium, being charged, is highly lipid-insoluble. Thus, ammonia readily diffuses across the renal cell membranes; whereas ammonium does not.

The synthesis of ammonia within the cell creates a cell-lumen concentration gradient down which ammonia diffuses. (Obviously, ammonia will diffuse into the blood also, but we ignore this for the sake of simplicity.) In both the cell and lumen, there exists an equilibrium between ammonia and ammonium. The key point is that the relative amounts of this buffer pair present in each phase depends upon pH. When the tubular fluid is acid, what happens to the ammonia after it diffuses into the lumen? Immediately, almost all of the ammonia combines with hydrogen ion to form ammonium. Thus, the ammonium concentration in the lumen increases, but since the membrane is virtually impermeable to ammonium, it is trapped within the lumen. Since the ammonia is converted to ammonium almost as fast as it enters, the concentration of ammonia in the lumen is kept low, and the concentration gradient from cell to lumen is maintained. Thus, ammonia passively diffuses into the lumen and is trapped there by conversion to ammonium. The lower the pH of the tubular fluid, the more effective this process, and the more ammonia that enters the lumen. It should be clear, therefore, that this process forces an efficient coupling between renal tubular acid secretion and the supply of buffer (ammonia) required to react with the secreted hydrogen ion. As the pH of the tubular fluid decreases because of increased acid secretion, the falling pH automatically induces increased entry and trapping of ammonia in the lumen with subsequent buffering of the hydrogen ions. As long as ammonia synthesis by the cells can keep up with demand (i.e., unbuffered hydrogen ions in the lumen), then hydrogen-ion secretion can continue without causing the tubular pH to reach the minimal limiting value. The fact that increased ammonia synthesis occurs during chronic acidosis (the adaptation process described above) permits ammonia to serve as the major urinary buffer in the kidneys' compensation for acidosis. Ammonium excretion may increase from a normal value of 20 mEq/day to 500 mEq/day in a person suffering from severe acidosis. In contrast, phosphate's contribution may increase by only 20 to 40 mEq/day.

The other side of this coin should also be emphasized: When the urine is not acid, there will be very little diffusion trapping of ammonia. Unless enough acid is secreted by the tubules to force a significant reduction of tubular-fluid pH, little ammonium will be excreted in the urine.

The process of diffusion trapping described above applies not only to ammonia but to the renal handling of many weak organic acids and bases which can exist in both the nonionized or ionized forms. For example, the excretion of the weak base quinine is markedly increased when the urine is highly acid. This is because nonionized quinine diffuses from the peritubular plasma and into the tubular lumen, where it is trapped by being converted in the acid tubular fluid to its ionized form. Note that this is really a form of passive tubular secretion.

QUALITATIVE INTEGRATION OF BICARBONATE REABSORPTION AND ACID EXCRETION

To reiterate, acid secreted by the tubules can suffer one of two general fates: (1) It can combine with filtered bicarbonate, in which case the overall process accomplishes bicarbonate reabsorption. (2) Or it can combine with filtered nonbicarbonate buffers such as phosphate or with ammonia that has been synthesized and secreted by the tubules.

The first case is a conservation process by which the kidneys prevent loss of bicarbonate from the body. This process alone does not alkalinize the body but rather prevents the development of an acidosis due to bicarbonate loss. In contrast, the second process contributes new bicarbonate to the body and simultaneously excretes acid, thereby alkalinizing it.

What determines whether the secreted hydrogen ions, once in the lumen, combine with bicarbonate, on the one hand, or with phosphate, ammonia, or organic buffers, on the other? This depends upon the pK's of each buffer-pair reaction and upon the mass of each buffer present. To simplify matters, one may assume that very little nonbicarbonate buffer is titrated, i.e., combines with hydrogen ion, until most of the bicarbonate has been reabsorbed. This phenomenon occurs largely because the quantity of bicarbonate is huge compared to the quantity of the other buffers. Once most of the filtered bicarbonate has been reabsorbed, then almost all of the secreted acid combines with the other buffers.

One can imagine, then, a spectrum of events reflecting the acid-base status of the body:

Alkalosis

When an alkalosis exists, the kidneys compensate by secreting too little acid to accomplish complete reabsorption of filtered bicarbonate. Therefore, bicarbonate is excreted in an alkaline urine, and the body is thereby made more acid. Simultaneously, because the acid secreted is inadequate to reabsorb all the bicarbonate, there is virtually no hydrogen ion available to combine with nonbicarbonate buffers. This is just what one would expect, teleologically, since the kidneys are "attempting" to eliminate bicarbonate from the body, not add new bicarbonate to it.

Normal State

Metabolism of the average American diet results in the net liberation of 40 to 80 mEq of hydrogen ion per day. Therefore, if balance is to be maintained, the kidneys must excrete this same amount of acid, i.e., contribute 40 to 80 mEq of new bicarbonate to the blood (again, we emphasize that these are synonymous statements). Accordingly, tubular acid secretion must be great enough to effect complete reabsorption of all filtered bicarbonate, and an additional 40 to 80 mEq acid must be secreted to contribute 40 to 80 mEq new bicarbonate to the blood, this acid being excreted in the urine buffered by phosphate and ammonia. The urine under such circumstances is moderately acid, perhaps at pH 6.

Acidosis

The kidneys compensate for acidosis by adding large quantities of new bicarbonate to the blood. Therefore, as in the previously described normal state, acid secretion must be great enough to effect complete reabsorption of all filtered bicarbonate. Beyond this, the tubules must secrete large amounts of additional acid so as to add an equivalent amount of new bicarbonate to the blood. This acid is excreted in the urine buffered by phosphate and ammonia and by organic buffers, when they are present. Under such conditions, ammonia becomes the most important buffer; its supply by diffusion trapping is assured by the fact that once all the bicarbonate is reabsorbed, the large continued secretion of acid causes the tubular-fluid pH to fall progressively.

It should now be clear how, via changes in the rate of a single variable, namely, the rate of tubular acid secretion, the kidneys can compensate for the entire range of acid-base patterns which can occur. The factors which regulate this process in response to acid-base changes will be discussed after the following section detailing the methods for *quantitating* renal handling of hydrogen ion.

QUANTITATION OF RENAL ACID-BASE FUNCTIONS

Measurement of Tubular Acid-secretion Rate

A hydrogen ion secreted by the tubules can combine in the lumen with bicarbonate, phosphate, or ammonia or with one of several organic buffers. In order to calculate the total mass of acid secreted per unit time, one must add up the contributions of all these pathways. The amount of free hydrogen ion may be ignored because it is so small.

It is worthwhile to emphasize once more the great difference between the fate of a hydrogen ion reacting with bicarbonate and the fate of one reacting with any of the other buffers. As described above, the combination of a hydrogen ion with bicarbonate causes the generation of carbon dioxide and water, both of which are reabsorbed by the tubules. Thus, the secreted hydrogen ion that is used for bicarbonate reabsorption does not remain in the urine. How, then, can one measure it? The answer depends upon the fact that one bicarbonate ion is reabsorbed as a result of the secretion of one hydrogen ion. Therefore, assuming this one-to-one ratio, we can calculate the mass of secreted hydrogen ion reacting with bicarbonate by measuring the rate of bicarbonate reabsorption. The rate is equal to the difference between filtered and excreted bicarbonate. For example, given the following data, how much secreted acid combined in the lumen with bicarbonate?

$$GFR = 180 \text{ liters/day}$$
$$P_{HCO_3^-} = 24 \text{ mEq/liter}$$
$$\text{Urine vol} = 1 \text{ liter/day}$$
$$U_{HCO_3^-} = 24 \text{ mEq/liter}$$
$$\text{Filtered } HCO_3^-/\text{day} = GFR \times P_{HCO_3^-}$$
$$= 180 \text{ liters/day} \times 24 \text{ mEq/liter}$$
$$= 4{,}320 \text{ mEq/day}$$
$$\text{Excreted } HCO_3^-/\text{day} = U_{HCO_3^-} \times V$$
$$= 24 \text{ mEq/liter} \times 1 \text{ liter/day}$$
$$= 24 \text{ mEq/day}$$
$$\text{Reabsorbed } HCO_3^-/\text{day} = \text{filtered } HCO_3^-/\text{day} - \text{excreted } HCO_3^-/\text{day}$$
$$= 4{,}320 \text{ mEq/day} - 24 \text{ mEq/day}$$
$$= 4{,}296 \text{ mEq/day}$$

Thus, 4,296 mEq H^+ must have been secreted to accomplish the reabsorption of 4,296 mEq HCO_3^-.

In contrast to the hydrogen ion which reacts with bicarbonate, that which combines with phosphate or organic buffers does remain in the tubular fluid and is excreted in the urine bound to the buffers. This quantity of acid can be measured by taking a sample of urine and titrating it with sodium hydroxide back to a pH of 7.4, the pH of the plasma from which the glomerular filtrate originated. This simply reverses the events which occurred within the tubular lumen when the tubular fluid was titrated by secreted hydrogen ions. Thus, the number of milliequivalents of sodium hydroxide required to reach pH 7.40 must equal the number of milliequivalents of hydrogen ion added to the tubular fluid which combined with phosphate and the organic buffers. This value is known as the *titratable acid*.

It must be stressed that the titratable-acid measurement does *not* pick up hydrogen ions which combined with ammonia to yield ammonium. The reason is that the pK of the ammonia-ammonium reaction is so high (9.2) that titration with alkali to pH 7.4 will not remove the hydrogen ions from the ammonium. In addition to measuring titratable acid, therefore, a separate measurement of urinary ammonium excretion must be performed.

The total rate of tubular hydrogen-ion secretion is thus equal to the sum of:

HCO_3^- reabsorption, mEq/time
+ titratable acid, mEq/time
+ NH_4^+ excretion, mEq/time

Values for a person on a normal diet are approximately:

HCO_3^- reabsorption = 4,300 mEq/day
Titratable acid = 20 mEq/day
NH_4^+ excretion = 40 mEq/day

These values serve to emphasize that the vast majority of secreted hydrogen ions are used to accomplish bicarbonate reabsorption, with only a small number remaining for the production of titratable acid or ammonium.

**Measurement of Renal Contribution
of New Bicarbonate
to the Blood**

The above analysis also indicates how to calculate the amount of new bicarbonate added to the blood by the kidneys, an extremely important number since it is a precise measure of the degree to which the kidneys have alkalinized the body. It is simply the sum of titratable acid and ammonium. This sum measures the rate of acid *excreted* in the urine secondary to tubular acid secretion, and, as we have stressed several times, it is identical to the quantity of new bicarbonate added by the renal tubular cells to the blood. This stems from the fact that each hydrogen ion secreted into the lumen which reacts with a nonbicarbonate buffer remains in the tubular fluid and is excreted.

We can now state the data required for a quantitative assessment of the renal contribution to acid-base regulation in any patient:

1. Titratable acid excreted	= new HCO_3^- added to the blood
2. + NH_4^+ excreted	= new HCO_3^- added to the blood
3. − HCO_3^- excreted	= unreabsorbed filtered HCO_3^- lost from the body because of incomplete reabsorption

Total = net HCO_3^- gain or loss to the body (negative values equal loss, positive values equal gain).

Typical urine data for the renal compensations in the three states described are as follows:

Alkalosis

$$\begin{array}{r}
\text{Titratable acid} = 0 \text{ mEq/day} \\
+ \text{NH}_4^+ = 0 \text{ mEq/day} \\
- \text{HCO}_3^- \text{ excreted} = -80 \text{ mEq/day} \\
\hline
80 \text{ mEq HCO}_3^- \text{ lost from the body} \\
(\text{Urine pH} = 8.0)
\end{array}$$

Normal state

$$\begin{array}{r}
\text{Titratable acid} = 20 \text{ mEq/day} \\
+ \text{NH}_4^+ = 40 \text{ mEq/day} \\
- \text{HCO}_3^- \text{ excreted} = -1 \text{ m Eq/day} \\
\hline
59 \text{ mEq HCO}_3^- \text{ added to the body} \\
(\text{Urine pH} = 6.0)
\end{array}$$

Acidosis

$$\begin{array}{r}
\text{Titratable acid} = 40 \text{ mEq/day} \\
+ \text{NH}_4^+ = 160 \text{ mEq/day} \\
- \text{HCO}_3^- \text{ excreted} = 0 \text{ mEq/day} \\
\hline
200 \text{ mEq HCO}_3^- \text{ added to the body} \\
(\text{Urine pH} = 4.6)
\end{array}$$

Note, however, that the data shown for alkalosis are typical for respiratory alkalosis and for "pure" metabolic alkalosis, i.e., alkalosis uncomplicated by other electrolyte abnormalities. As we shall see in subsequent sections, other electrolyte imbalances frequently complicate the picture in metabolic alkalosis so that the urine may not be alkaline.

CONTROL OF RENAL TUBULAR ACID SECRETION

There are multiple factors which control the key element in the kidneys' acid-base machinery, the rate of tubular acid secretion. Several of these factors control acid secretion so as to homeostatically regulate the pH of the body fluids. Others, which reflect the balances of sodium, chloride, and potassium in the body, influence acid secretion not as a part of pH-regulating reflexes but rather because the transport of each of these substances is interrelated with the transport of the others (see below).

Glomerulotubular Balance for Bicarbonate

One of the important influences on hydrogen secretion is analogous to the phenomenon of glomerulotubular balance previously described for sodium. Hydrogen secretion (and, therefore, bicarbonate reabsorption) varies directly with GFR. For example, if GFR increases 25 percent, so does bicarbonate reabsorption. The adaptive value of such a relationship is that changes in GFR do not induce potentially serious perturbations in the acid-base status of the body. (Note that changes in GFR are usually reflexly elicited in response to extracellular-volume changes, not in response to acid-base changes.) In the example of the 25-percent increase cited above, if acid secretion and bicarbonate reabsorption did not increase proportionally to GFR, a very large quantity of bicarbonate would be lost from the body with a resulting acidosis. The mechanism responsible for bicarbonate glomerulotubular balance is not clear at present.

Pco_2 and Renal Intracellular pH

The most important single determinant of the rate of tubular acid secretion is the Pco_2 of the arterial blood. As shown in Fig. 33, the rate of hydrogen-ion secretion, as manifested by bicarbonate reabsorptive rate, is directly related to the Pco_2 of the arterial plasma. (In this figure, bicarbonate reabsorption is expressed in milliequivalents per liter GFR rather than in milliequivalents per time because of the previously described influence of glomerulotubular balance.) This relationship holds over the entire range of arterial Pco_2 values.

There are no nerves or hormones mediating this response; rather, the renal tubular cells respond to the Pco_2 of the blood perfusing them.

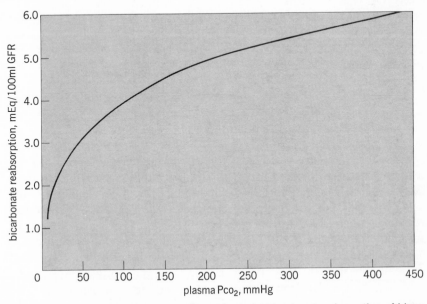

Figure 33 The relationship between Pco_2 of arterial blood and reabsorption of bicarbonate in the dog. [*Data from F. C. Rector, Jr., et al., J. Clin. Invest.,* **39**:1706 (1960).]

An increased P_{CO_2} of arterial blood causes, by diffusion of carbon dioxide, an equivalent increase in P_{CO_2} within the tubular cells. This causes an increased rate of formation of carbonic acid and, in turn, an elevated intracellular hydrogen-ion concentration. Presumably, it is this change that directly stimulates the rate of hydrogen-ion secretion. In other words, the ultimate stimulus for hydrogen-ion secretion is not the P_{CO_2}, per se, but rather the decreased intracellular pH it induces.

The reason that intracellular pH is so responsive to changes in arterial P_{CO_2} is the ease with which carbon dioxide diffuses across cell membranes. Thus, a small change in blood P_{CO_2} causes an almost immediate equivalent change in cell P_{CO_2} which, by mass action, alters cell pH. In contrast to this sensitivity to P_{CO_2} changes, cell pH is much less dependent upon changes in blood pH, per se — the reasons being that cell membranes are less permeable to the diffusion of hydrogen ion itself (or of bicarbonate) and that active-transport mechanisms for hydrogen ion can minimize the transmission of extracellular pH changes into the cell. This is not to say that the cells are completely impervious to extracellular pH changes unaccompanied by simultaneous changes in P_{CO_2}. Such extracellular pH changes generally do influence intracellular pH but much less than extracellular P_{CO_2} changes do. Accordingly, the rate of renal acid secretion correlates better with blood P_{CO_2} than with blood pH.

Renal Compensation for Respiratory Acidosis and Alkalosis

Let us apply this analysis to the clinical situations respiratory acidosis and alkalosis. For reference, we shall present the basic equations again (CO_2 rather than H_2CO_3 can be used in the second equation because the concentrations are always in direct proportion to one another):

$$H_2O + CO_2 \rightleftharpoons H_2CO_3 \rightleftharpoons H^+ + HCO_3^-$$

$$[H^+] = K \frac{[CO_2]}{[HCO_3^-]}$$

In chronic pulmonary insufficiency, carbon dioxide is retained, and the resulting increase in P_{CO_2} drives the carbon dioxide–bicarbonate reaction to the right with a resulting acidosis. It should be clear from both equations that the pH could be restored to normal if the bicarbonate could be elevated to the same degree as the P_{CO_2}. There is, of course, an automatic increase in bicarbonate concentration solely as a result of the reaction being driven to the right, but this is not nearly to the same degree as the rise in P_{CO_2}. If we rewrite the equation, we can see why mass action does not lead to proportionate increases of bicarbonate and carbon dioxide:

$$[H^+][HCO_3^-] = K[CO_2]$$

Thus a rise in carbon dioxide causes a proportionate rise in the product $[H^+][HCO_3^-]$. Since hydrogen-ion concentration also increases, bicarbonate concentration cannot increase as much as carbon dioxide does.

It is the kidneys' job to cause the additional bicarbonate increase by contributing new bicarbonate to the blood. This occurs as a result of the increased P_{CO_2}, which stimulates renal tubular acid secretion so that all filtered bicarbonate is reabsorbed and much secreted acid is left over for the formation of titratable acid and ammonium, i.e., for the addition of new bicarbonate to the blood. This process continues until a new steady state is reached, at which point the plasma bicarbonate is now so high that even the enhanced rate of acid secretion can serve only to reabsorb the increased filtered load of bicarbonate and cannot contribute large amounts of new bicarbonate. The renal compensation is not usually perfect; i.e., when the steady state is reached, the plasma bicarbonate is not elevated to quite the same degree as the P_{CO_2} is. Consequently, blood pH is not completely returned to normal.

The sequence of events in response to respiratory alkalosis is just the opposite. As a result of hyperventilation, the patient transiently eliminates carbon dioxide faster than it is produced, thereby lowering his P_{CO_2} and raising plasma pH. The decreased P_{CO_2} reduces tubular acid secretion so that bicarbonate reabsorption is not complete. Bicarbonate is then lost from the body, and the loss results in a decreased plasma bicarbonate and a return toward normal pH.

**Renal Compensation for Metabolic
Acidosis and Alkalosis**

The primary cause of so-called metabolic acidosis is either the addition to the body (by ingestion, infusion, or production) of increased amounts of acid other than carbonic acid, or, alternatively, the loss from the body of bicarbonate (as in diarrhea). Inspection of the equations reveals that either loss of bicarbonate or addition of hydrogen ions will lower both the plasma pH and the plasma bicarbonate concentration. The kidney compensation is to raise the plasma bicarbonate concentration back toward normal, thereby returning pH toward normal. In order to do this, the kidneys must reabsorb all the filtered bicarbonate and contribute new bicarbonate through the formation of titratable acid and ammonium. This is precisely what normal kidneys do, and the urines excreted in respiratory and metabolic acidosis are indistinguishable in these respects.

Yet, the surprising fact is that, in metabolic acidosis (in contrast to respiratory acidosis), these events occur in the absence of a significant stimulus to the kidney to increase acid secretion; indeed, they frequently occur in the presence of a decreased stimulus. This is because, as described above, the P_{CO_2} of arterial blood, which is the major stimulus for tubular acid secretion, is *not increased* in metabolic acidosis but is usually *decreased*. Why? Because, as the arterial pH falls as a result of whatever is causing the metabolic acidosis, pulmonary ventilation is stimulated. This is, of course, the respiratory compensation for the acidosis and its effect is to reduce arterial P_{CO_2}. Therefore, because renal-tubular-cell pH is rapidly altered by changes in P_{CO_2}, renal-tubular-cell pH is likely to be increased in the early stages of metabolic acidosis. (In patients with chronic metabolic acidosis, it is likely that intracellular pH returns to normal or actually decreases despite a continued decrease in P_{CO_2}, probably because of altered peritubular-membrane transport of hydrogen ion.)

How, then, can the kidneys manage to perform their compensatory function with no stimulus to increase acid secretion? This apparent paradox is resolved when one recalls that in uncompensated metabolic acidosis the plasma bicarbonate is lower than normal (in contrast, during respiratory acidosis plasma bicarbonate is greater than normal, even in the uncompensated state). Therefore, the mass of bicarbonate filtered is reduced proportionally to the decreased plasma bicarbonate, and less hydrogen ion need be secreted to accomplish its total reabsorption. Accordingly, even with a decreased total acid secretion, there is still considerable hydrogen ion available after the bicarbonate has been completely reabsorbed to form large amounts of titratable acid and ammonium, i.e., to contribute new bicarbonate to the plasma. For example, compare the data for a person with metabolic acidosis with those for a normal person:

	Normal	*Metabolic acidosis*
Plasma HCO_3^-	24 mEq/liter	12 mEq/liter
GFR	180 liters/day	180 liters/day
Filtered HCO_3^-	4,320 mEq/day	2,160 mEq/day
1. Reabsorbed HCO_3^-	4,315 mEq/day	2,160 mEq/day
2. Titratable acid and NH_4^+	60 mEq/day	200 mEq/day
3. Total H^+ secreted [(1) + (2)]	4,375 mEq/day	2,360 mEq/day

Thus, even in the presence of a greatly reduced acid secretion, the kidneys are able to compensate for the metabolic acidosis. Indeed, the limiting factor in this type of acidosis turns out to be not the rate of acid secretion but rather the availability of buffer.

The situation in metabolic alkalosis is just the opposite; despite a normal or increased rate of acid secretion (secondary to a reflexly elevated P_{CO_2}) the load of filtered bicarbonate is so great that much bicarbonate escapes reabsorption and no titratable acid or ammonium can be formed. Therefore, plasma bicarbonate is decreased, and pH decreases toward normal.

This completes our discussion of the mechanisms by which hydrogen-ion secretion is controlled so as to achieve acid-base homeostasis. We now describe how factors not designed to maintain pH constant can also influence hydrogen-ion secretion and bicarbonate reabsorption so as to move pH away from normal. In other words, just as was true for potassium, hydrogen-ion balance has its own distinct homeostatic controls, but it is also at the mercy of other interacting events, the most important of which are extracellular-volume contraction and potassium depletion. Again, similarly to potassium, these interactions are the result of the close interlinking of sodium, potassium, chloride, and hydrogen-ion handling by the kidney.

Influence of Salt Depletion on Acid Secretion

The presence of salt depletion interferes with the ability of the kidneys to compensate for a metabolic alkalosis. In metabolic alkalosis, the plasma bicarbonate is elevated, either because of addition of bicarbonate to the body or because of loss of acid from it. The normal renal compensation should be to set hydrogen-ion secretion at a level which fails to achieve complete bicarbonate reabsorption and thereby allows the excess bicarbonate to be excreted. But when salt depletion is present simultaneously, a situation is created in which mutually exclusive demands are placed upon the tubule. On the one hand, the need for conservation of salt demands that the urine be virtually free of sodium, and to this end the usual sodium-retaining reflexes are triggered. On the other hand, the need for compensating the metabolic alkalosis demands that bicarbonate be excreted in the urine, but for this to occur, some cation (mainly sodium) must be excreted with the bicarbonate. In this conflict, the sodium-conserving reflexes are dominant, sodium reabsorption is complete, and no sodium appears in the urine. Therefore, almost no bicarbonate can appear either. What happens is that the presence of the salt depletion not only stimulates sodium reabsorption but also stimulates hydrogen-ion secretion so that virtually all the filtered bicarbonate is reabsorbed. (The actual mechanisms by which the salt depletion enhances hydrogen-ion secretion are unclear at present.) The net result is that the already elevated plasma bicarbonate associated with the metabolic alkalosis is locked in and the plasma pH remains unchanged; instead of being alkaline as it should, the urine is moderately acid.

It should be emphasized that salt depletion will not *cause* a metabolic alkalosis; rather, it merely reduces the ability of the kidneys to compensate for any metabolic alkalosis once the alkalosis is established.

The reason why salt depletion, per se, does not cause alkalosis is simple: If the plasma bicarbonate level is normal to start with, reabsorption of all the filtered bicarbonate along with sodium merely maintains the same normal plasma bicarbonate level. It does not increase plasma bicarbonate level. The situation is analogous to the reabsorption of glucose in normal individuals; i.e., reabsorption of all the filtered glucose merely keeps plasma glucose at the normal level.

Finally, it should be noted that we have referred to salt depletion in this section without distinguishing between sodium and chloride losses. This is because loss of either of these ions will lead to extracellular-volume contraction and the enhancement of sodium-retaining reflexes. (At present, however, there is considerable controversy concerning a possible specific, additional effect of chloride deficiency, but no clear-cut answer is available.)

Influence of Potassium Balance

Renal acid secretion and bicarbonate reabsorption are strongly influenced by the body's potassium balance. As a result, primary changes in potassium balance can produce secondary shifts of body-fluid hydrogen-ion balance away from normal. For example, a state of potassium depletion frequently stimulates tubular acid secretion, the result being the contribution of an abnormally large quantity of new bicarbonate to the body, thereby causing the development of a metabolic alkalosis. Note that there was nothing wrong with acid-base balance to start with; the alkalosis was caused by an oversecretion of acid by the kidneys because of potassium depletion. Conversely, a primary state of potassium retention may inhibit the normal rate of renal acid secretion resulting in the excretion of large amounts of bicarbonate in the urine and the development of a metabolic acidosis.

We have now come full circle. Recall from the section on renal handling of potassium that the acidity of the body fluids can have a strong influence on potassium balance by altering renal tubular potassium secretion. Now we see that the converse is also true. The most important of these relationships pertains to alkalosis and potassium depletion:

$$\text{Alkalosis} \rightarrow \ \uparrow K^+ \text{ secretion} \rightarrow K^+ \text{ depletion}$$
$$K^+ \text{ depletion} \rightarrow \ \uparrow \text{acid secretion} \rightarrow \text{alkalosis}$$

Note that these relationships constitute a positive-feedback cycle. Thus:

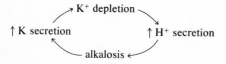

Of course, as potassium depletion progresses, specific homeostatic regulators of potassium secretion oppose the cycle. These regulators (particularly reduced tubular-cell concentration of potassium) will tend to impede further potassium secretion.[1]

What are the factors linking potassium depletion and alkalosis? The answer is intracellular pH and potassium concentration. We previously pointed out that the presence of an alkalosis increases intracellular potassium. As you might predict, the reciprocal relation also holds: Cell potassium depletion apparently causes a decrease in renal-cell pH; whereas an increased cell potassium induces increased cell pH. These influences are probably best explained by the ability of potassium and hydrogen ion to inhibit each other's transport across the renal peritubular membrane and into the tubular cells. This relationship is certainly not limited to the kidney; it also exists in many other cells of the body such as skeletal muscle.

Influence of Hydrogen-ion Secretion on Sodium Chloride Reabsorption

The previous section described how alterations in salt balance could influence hydrogen-ion secretion. This section deals with the reverse phenomenon, the ability of primary changes in hydrogen-ion secretion and bicarbonate reabsorption to alter sodium and chloride handling.

In describing the secretion of hydrogen ions along the nephron, it is frequently stated that secreted hydrogen ions are exchanged for sodium. It now seems clear that this exchange does not represent a coupled sodium–hydrogen-ion exchange pump as was once visualized. Rather it results from the fact that chloride and bicarbonate constitute the only quantitatively important anions in the glomerular filtrate and from the requirement that electroneutrality be maintained in the tubular lumen.

Visualize what happens in the proximal tubule. Sodium ions are reabsorbed actively, and this results in the passive reabsorption of chloride, so that electroneutrality is maintained. However, approximately one-sixth of the filtered sodium is associated with bicarbonate rather than with chloride. Therefore, unless the bicarbonate were reabsorbed at close to the same rate as this moiety of sodium is, there would occur a

---

[1] At present, considerable controversy exists concerning whether potassium deficiency, per se, can perturb acid-base balance as described above or whether the real culprit is extracellular-volume contraction, which frequently occurs along with potassium depletion. (Extracellular-volume contraction and potassium depletion may result from the same disease process, e.g., by vomiting.) We believe that present evidence warrants the conclusion that the effects of potassium depletion are, in fact, distinct and important, particularly when the depletion is quite severe. Moreover, it should also be noted that potassium deficiency can actually *induce* an alkalosis; whereas extracellular-volume contraction does not produce alkalosis *de novo* but rather prevents its repair by the kidneys. (See Seldin and Rector, 1972, in Suggested Readings for Chap. 8.)

large separation of charge and a marked increase in the negativity of the tubular lumen—an event which would strongly retard further net sodium reabsorption. In fact, bicarbonate reabsorption normally does occur at the same rate, or faster than, sodium; since the bicarbonate is reabsorbed as a result of hydrogen-ion secretion, there is, in a sense, the exchange of a secreted hydrogen ion for a reabsorbed sodium ion, although the active-transport systems are distinct (Fig. 34).

This type of exchange occurs not only when the secreted hydrogen ion achieves bicarbonate reabsorption but also when the hydrogen ion is used in the formation of titratable acid and ammonium. Note (Fig. 35) that in both cases the titration of HPO_4^{2-} to $H_2PO_4^-$ or of NH_3 to NH_4^+ produces a net gain of one positive charge in the lumen, thereby permitting a sodium ion to be reabsorbed simultaneously with no change in intraluminal charge.

In effect, then, sodium is reabsorbed either with chloride or in exchange for hydrogen ion. There are several very important implications of these relationships for sodium chloride reabsorption.

(1) There is usually an inverse correlation between the excretion rates of chloride and bicarbonate. Most simply viewed, when sodium reabsorption is proceeding relatively more rapidly than acid secretion and bicarbonate reabsorption is, then more chloride will accompany the reabsorbed sodium. Therefore, as a result of electrical events within the tubules, less chloride will be excreted. Conversely, when the rate of acid secretion is high enough so that filtrated bicarbonate is totally reabsorbed and large quantities of titratable acid and ammonium are formed, then less chloride is reabsorbed since a larger fraction of the sodium is reabsorbed in exchange for hydrogen ion. Thus, the net effect of these latter events, which occur in response to acidosis, is to reduce plasma chloride while simultaneously increasing plasma bicarbonate.

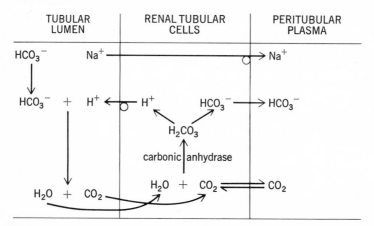

Figure 34 Tubular sodium-hydrogen exchange during reabsorption of bicarbonate.

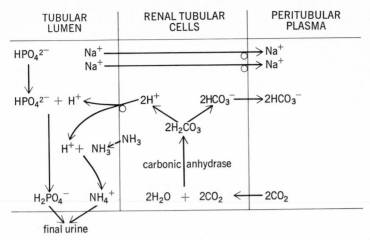

| TUBULAR LUMEN | RENAL TUBULAR CELLS | PERITUBULAR PLASMA |

Figure 35 Tubular sodium-hydrogen ion exchange during formation of titratable acid and ammonium.

(2) Whenever tubular acid secretion is inadequate to effect complete bicarbonate reabsorption, there is usually the obligatory excretion of some sodium in the urine along with the bicarbonate. However, the loss of sodium is usually not as great as the loss of bicarbonate, because alkalosis also induces increased potassium secretion, as described above, and the secretion of potassium ions into the lumen allows an equivalent amount of sodium to be reabsorbed with no change in intraluminal potential. An interesting example of this phenomenon is the renal response to administration of drugs which inhibit renal carbonic anhydrase. Inhibition of this enzyme reduces acid secretion, which in turn reduces bicarbonate reabsorption. The net result is an increased excretion of sodium, bicarbonate, and water. (Unreabsorbed solute always causes the excretion of increased amounts of water.) In addition, the inhibition of carbonic anhydrase alkalinizes the renal tubular cells. The increased intracellular pH induces an enhanced secretion of potassium so that a large fraction of the excreted bicarbonate is accompanied by potassium rather than by sodium.

Study questions: **40** to **45**

Chapter 9

Regulation of Calcium Balance and Extracellular Concentration

OBJECTIVES

The student understands the regulation of calcium balance and extracellular concentration.

1 States the normal plasma calcium concentration and the percent which is protein-bound; states the effect of pH on the free fraction
2 Lists the effector sites for calcium homeostasis and the effects of parathormone, vitamin D, and calcitonin on them
3 Describes the origin and control of secretion rates of parathormone and calcitonin
4 Describes the origins of vitamin D and controls over its activity
5 Describes the relationships between parathormone and vitamin D
6 Describes the direct and indirect effects of an increased plasma calcium concentration on renal calcium handling
7 Predicts changes in plasma and urinary calcium and phosphate in a patient with hyperparathyroidism; also in a patient with vitamin D deficiency

Extracellular calcium concentration is normally maintained within very narrow limits, the requirement for precise regulation stemming primarily from the profound effects of calcium on neuromuscular excitability. A low calcium concentration increases the excitability of nerve and muscle cell membranes so that patients with diseases in which low calcium occurs suffer from *hypocalcemic tetany,* characterized by skeletal muscle spasms which can be severe enough to cause death by asphyxia. Calcium is also important in blood clotting, but low calcium is never clinically a cause of abnormal clotting because the levels required for this function are considerably below those which produce fatal tetany. Hypercalcemia is also dangerous, because it causes cardiac arrhythmias as well as depressed neuromuscular excitability.

It is important to recognize that the plasma calcium (normally 5 mEq/liter or 2.5 mmol/liter) is approximately 50-percent protein-bound. Since only the free, i.e., ionized, calcium exerts effects on nerve, muscle, and other target organs, any factor which influences the degree of protein binding can increase or decrease the effects of calcium. One of the most important influences on binding is the plasma pH. An increase in pH causes increased calcium binding, because the decreased acidity converts more of the protein to the anionic form; i.e., it exposes additional negatively charged binding sites. Thus, a patient with alkalosis is extremely susceptible to tetany; whereas a patient with acidosis will not manifest tetany at levels of total plasma calcium low enough to cause symptoms in normal people.

EFFECTOR SITES FOR CALCIUM HOMEOSTASIS

Our earlier sections on ion and water homeostasis were concerned almost entirely with the renal handling of these substances. It was possible to do so for several reasons: (1) Although internal exchanges (between extracellular fluid, on the one hand, and bone and cells, on the other) are important for these substances, the major homeostatic controls act via the kidneys. (2) Absorption of these substances from the gut approximates 100 percent under normal circumstances and is not a major controlled variable. Neither of these statements holds true for calcium homeostasis. Accordingly, this section must deal not only with the renal handling of calcium but with the other two major effector sites for calcium homeostasis — bone and the gastrointestinal tract.

Gastrointestinal Tract

The gastrointestinal tract indiscriminately absorbs virtually the total quantity of many ingested substances. But this is not true for calcium absorption, whose active-transport system is subject to quite precise hormonal control. Normally, the *net* absorption of calcium amounts to only 10 percent of that ingested, the remainder being excreted in the feces.

However, the situation is complex, since the intestinal epithelium secretes considerable amounts of endogenous calcium into the lumen.

$$
\begin{array}{rl}
\text{Ca ingested} =& 1{,}000 \text{ mg/day} \\
\text{Ca secreted into intestinal lumen} =& \underline{600 \text{ mg/day}} \\
\text{Total in intestinal lumen} =& 1{,}600 \text{ mg/day} \\
\text{Absorbed from gut} =& \underline{700 \text{ mg/day}} \\
\text{Excreted in feces} =& 900 \text{ mg/day}
\end{array}
$$

In this example, 100 mg of new calcium is added to the blood each day, i.e., 10 percent of the ingested calcium. Note, however, that if gut absorption were reduced to 600 mg/day, then none of the ingested calcium would have been retained. Conversely, retention could potentially be increased tenfold were absorption raised to 1,600 mg/day. Finally, lowering the rate of absorption to 500 mg/day would result in the fecal loss of 1,100 mg/day; i.e., the person would go into negative calcium balance. As we shall see, control of gut calcium absorption constitutes an important homeostatic mechanism for regulating total body balance and extracellular concentration.

Kidney

The kidneys handle calcium by filtration and reabsorption. Only 50 percent of the plasma calcium is filterable, the remainder being protein-bound. The reabsorption process is active, occurs throughout the nephron, and normally approximates 99 percent. The 1 percent which escapes reabsorption amounts to approximately 100 mg/day, a quantity equal to the normal net addition of new calcium to the body via the gastrointestinal tract. Thus, just as was true for the other ions discussed in this book, the kidneys help maintain a constant balance of total body calcium by matching output to intake. When net intake is altered, the rate of excretion is homeostatically altered so as to maintain the balance.

Since calcium is filtered and reabsorbed, but not secreted:

$$\text{Ca excretion} = \text{Ca filtered} - \text{Ca reabsorbed}$$

Accordingly, excretion can be altered homeostatically by changing either the filtered load or the rate of reabsorption. Both occur. For example, what happens when a person increases his calcium intake? Transiently, intake exceeds output, positive calcium balance ensues, and plasma calcium concentration increases. This, in itself, increases the filtered mass of calcium (filtered $Ca = GFR \times P_{Ca}$) and increases excretion. Simultaneously, as we shall see, the increased plasma calcium triggers hormonal changes which cause a diminished reabsorption; i.e., it triggers decreased secretion of parathyroid hormone. The net result of these responses is increased calcium excretion and a restoration of balance.

These two mechanisms appear to be well established and important factors, but it is likely that others exist as well. Moreover, calcium reabsorption is also influenced by a large number of other ions (sodium, in particular) and by other hormones. The interested reader should consult the Suggested Readings.

Bone

The activities of the gastrointestinal tract and the kidneys determine the net intake and output of calcium for the entire body and, thereby, the overall state of calcium balance. In contrast, interchanges of calcium between extracellular fluid and bone do not alter total body balance but, rather, the distribution of calcium within the body. Approximately 99 percent of the total body calcium is contained in bone, which is basically a collagen-protein framework upon which calcium phosphate (and other minerals) are deposited in a crystal structure known as *hydroxyapatite*. Bone is not at all a dead, fixed tissue; rather, it is quite cellular and well supplied with blood. Most important, it is continuously broken down (resorbed) under the influence of cells called *osteoclasts* and simultaneously reformed under the influence of a different cell group called *osteoblasts*. The mechanisms by which these opposing processes occur are not completely understood, but at least one important factor seems to be the solubility product of calcium phosphate. An ionic compound will precipitate out of solution whenever the product of the concentrations of the individual ions exceeds a fixed value known as the solubility product. Thus, when calcium and/or phosphate concentrations increase so that $[Ca^{2+}][PO_4^{3-}]$ exceeds the solubility product, calcium phosphate precipitates out; this may occur locally at various sites in bone under the influence of enzymes secreted by bone cells. For example, osteoblasts produce the enzyme alkaline phosphatase, which catalyzes the splitting of various phosphate esters, thereby elevating the local concentration of free phosphate: As a result, $[Ca^{2+}][PO_4^{3-}]$ exceeds the solubility product, the minerals crystallize on to the organic matrix, and new bone is formed. Regardless of the precise mechanisms, the fact is that bone provides a huge potential source or sink for the withdrawal or deposit of calcium from extracellular fluid. We shall see that several hormones exert important effects on the deposition or resorption of bone calcium.

HORMONAL CONTROL OF EFFECTOR SITES

Parathormone

All three of the effector sites described above are subject to control by a protein hormone called parathormone (also called parathyroid hormone),

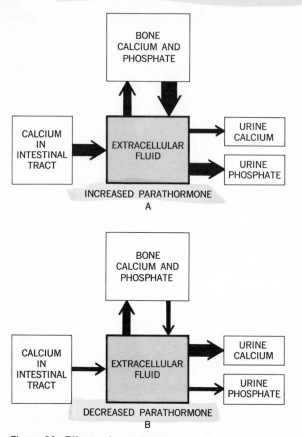

Figure 36   Effects of parathormone on the gastrointestinal tract, kidneys, and bone; the arrows signify relative magnitudes. Note that, when parathormone is decreased, there is net movement of calcium and phosphate into bone, urine calcium is raised, and gastrointestinal absorption of calcium is reduced. (*From A. J. Vander et al., "Human Physiology," © 1970 by McGraw-Hill, Inc. Used with permission of McGraw-Hill Book Company.*)

produced by the parathyroid glands. Parathormone production is controlled directly by the calcium concentration of the extracellular fluid bathing the cells of these glands. Lower calcium concentration stimulates parathormone production and release, and a higher concentration does just the opposite. It should be emphasized that extracellular calcium concentration acts directly upon the parathyroids without any intermediary hormones or nerves. (Recall that this is also true of the relation between extracellular potassium and aldosterone production.)

Parathormone exerts at least four distinct effects on the effector sites described earlier (Fig. 36):

1   It increases the movement of calcium (and phosphate) from bone into extracellular fluid by stimulating the osteoclasts, which break down bone structure, and thus liberating calcium phosphate crystals. In this manner the immense store of calcium contained in bone is made available for the regulation of extracellular calcium concentration.

2 It increases gastrointestinal absorption of calcium by stimulating the active-transport system which moves the ion from gut lumen to blood.

3 It increases renal tubular calcium reabsorption and thus decreases urinary calcium excretion.

4 It reduces the renal tubular reabsorption of phosphate and thereby raises urinary phosphate excretion and lowers extracellular phosphate concentration.

The adaptive value of the first three effects should be obvious: They all result in a higher extracellular calcium concentration and thus compensate for the lower concentration, which originally stimulated parathormone production. The adaptive value of the fourth effect requires further explanation and is a function of the $[Ca^{2+}][PO_4^{3-}]$ solubility product. Because of the solubility characteristics of undissociated calcium phosphate, the product of the extracellular concentrations of calcium and phosphate is approximately a constant. In other words, if the extracellular concentration of phosphate increases, it forces the deposition of some extracellular calcium in bone. This lowers the calcium concentration and keeps the calcium phosphate product a constant. The converse is also true. Imagine now what happens when parathormone causes the breakdown of bone. Both calcium and phosphate are released into the extracellular fluid. If the phosphate concentration were allowed to increase, further movement of calcium from bone would be retarded. But in addition to this effect on bone, we have seen that parathormone also decreases tubular reabsorption of phosphate and thus permits the excess phosphate to be eliminated in the urine. Indeed, extracellular phosphate is actually reduced by this mechanism, which allows even more calcium to be mobilized from bone.

In contrast to the state described above, an increase in extracellular calcium concentration inhibits normal parathormone production and thereby produces increased urinary and fecal calcium loss and net movement of calcium from extracellular fluid into bone (Fig. 36B).

Parathormone has other functions in the body, notably its role in milk production, but the four effects discussed above constitute the major mechanisms by which it integrates various organs and tissues in the regulation of extracellular calcium concentration.

Hyperparathyroidism, due to a primary defect in the parathyroid glands (e.g., a parathormone-secreting tumor), well illustrates the actions of parathormone. The excess hormone causes enhanced bone resorption leading to bone thinning with the formation of completely calcium-free areas or cysts. Plasma calcium increases and plasma phosphate decreases; the latter is caused by increased phosphate excretion. The increased plasma calcium is deposited in various body tissues including the kidneys, where stones are formed. A seeming paradox is that calcium excretion is increased. This occurs despite the fact that tubular calcium reabsorption is enhanced by parathormone. The explanation is that, because of the elevated plasma calcium, the filtered load of calcium increases even more than does reabsorptive rate—another excellent illustration of the necessity of taking both filtration and reabsorption into account when analyzing excretory changes.

Vitamin D

Vitamin D plays an important role in calcium metabolism, as attested by the fact that its deficiency results in poorly calcified bones. The term vitamin D denotes a group of closely related sterols. One of these compounds, now called vitamin D_3, is formed by the action of ultraviolet radiation on a provitamin (7-dehydrocholesterol) in the skin. Vitamin D_3 enters the blood and is hydroxylated several times, first by the liver and then by the kidneys, to the active form of the vitamin D sterols. From this description, it should be evident that the vitamin D formed in this way is actually a hormone, not a vitamin, since it is made in the body. However, man, because of his clothing and decreased out-of-doors life, is usually dependent upon dietary vitamin D for much of his supply. This dietary vitamin D must undergo the same hepatic and renal activation as does the vitamin D_3 produced in the skin.

The major action of vitamin D is to stimulate active calcium absorption by the intestine. It is of greater importance in this regard than parathormone; indeed, the action of parathormone is, itself, dependent upon the presence of adequate quantities of vitamin D. Thus, the major event in vitamin D deficiency is decreased gut calcium absorption resulting in decreased plasma calcium. In children, the newly formed bone protein matrix fails to be calcified normally because of the low plasma calcium, leading to the disease *rickets*.

In addition to its effect on intestinal calcium absorption, vitamin D also significantly enhances bone resorption. The mechanism underlying this effect is unclear but seems to involve a facilitation by vitamin D of the bone-resorption effect exerted by parathormone. Thus, in at least two of its actions (stimulation of gut absorption and bone resorption) parathormone is dependent for its full effect upon the simultaneous presence of adequate amounts of vitamin D.

The blood concentration of active vitamin D is subject to physiological control. The major control point is the final hydroxylation step, which occurs in the kidneys. This step is stimulated by parathormone. This is, of course, highly adaptive, for it provides an additional mechanism for simultaneously increasing or decreasing the levels of these closely interacting mediators. Thus a low plasma concentration stimulates the secretion of parathormone, which, in turn, enhances the activation of vitamin D, and both substances contribute to the restoration of the plasma calcium to normal.[1]

Calcitonin

Another hormone, calcitonin (also known as thyrocalcitonin), has significant effects on plasma calcium. Calcitonin is secreted by cells within the thyroid gland which surround, but are completely distinct from, the thyroxine-secreting follicles. The calcitonin-secreting cells are called, therefore, *parafollicular cells*. Calcitonin lowers plasma calcium primarily by inhibiting bone breakdown. Its secretion is controlled directly by the calcium concentration of the plasma supplying the thyroid gland; an increased calcium causes increased calcitonin secretion. Thus, this system constitutes a second important feedback control over plasma calcium concentration, one that is opposed to the parathormone system. However, its overall contribution to calcium homeostasis is minor compared to that of parathormone.

Other Hormones

Parathormone, calcitonin, and vitamin D are the only hormones whose production rates are altered as part of homeostatic responses to calcium balance. However, several other hormones do influence calcium, so that changes in their rates of secretion can produce calcium imbalances. Thus, high levels of cortisol can induce negative calcium balance by depressing gut absorption of calcium while increasing its renal excretion. Growth hormone also increases urinary calcium excretion, but it simultaneously increases gut absorption. The net effect of these counterbalancing influences of growth hormone is usually a positive calcium balance.

Study question: **46**

---

[1] The ability of parathormone to stimulate the activation of vitamin D may account for parathormone's action on gut calcium absorption; this effect is probably not *directly* due to parathormone but rather is mediated by the vitamin D increase caused by parathormone. Such is consistent with the fact, mentioned earlier, that the gut response to parathormone requires the presence of vitamin D.

Study Questions

1 True or False. The difference between superficial and juxtamedullary nephrons is that the former have their glomeruli in the cortex whereas the glomeruli of the latter arise in the medulla.

False. All glomeruli are in the cortex. See text for description.

2 Vitamin T is present in the urine. Does this *prove* that it is filterable at the glomerulus?

No. It is a possibility, but there is another; vitamin T may be secreted by the tubules.

3 Vitamin O is filtered, reabsorbed, and secreted. If you were designing a system for increasing the renal excretion of vitamin O

There are three possibilities (either alone or in combination): Increase filtered vitamin O by increasing either GFR or plasma concentra-

when its intake is high, what could you do?

tion of vitamin O; inhibit tubular reabsorption of vitamin O; enhance tubular secretion of vitamin O.

4   A drug is given which dilates the afferent arterioles. What happens to GFR?

It increases because of an increased glomerular-capillary pressure.

5   If the concentration of protein in the glomerular filtrate was 0.005 gm/100 ml and none was reabsorbed, how much protein would be excreted per day (assuming a normal GFR)?

9 gm.

Excreted
$$= \text{filtered} - \text{reabsorbed}$$
$$= (0.05 \text{ gm/liter}$$
$$\times 180 \text{ liters/day}) - 0$$
$$= 9 \text{ gm/day}$$

6   The hospital lab reports that your patient's creatinine clearance is 120 gm/day. This value is:
  a   Normal
  b   Significantly below normal
  c   Nonsense

c. Clearance units are volume per time, not mass per time.

7   The following test results were obtained on specimens from a person over a 24-hr period.

Total urine vol = 1.4 liters
$U_{In} = 100 \text{ mg/100 ml}$
$P_{In} = 1 \text{ mg/100 ml}$
$U_{urea} = 220 \text{ mmol/liter}$
$P_{urea} = 5 \text{ mmol/liter}$
$U_{PAH} = 700 \text{ mg/ml}$
$P_{PAH} = 2 \text{ mg/ml}$
Hematocrit = 0.40

What are the clearances of inulin, urea, and PAH? What is the effective renal plasma flow (ERPF)? What is the effective renal blood flow (ERBF)? How much urea is reabsorbed? How much PAH is secreted (assuming no PAH reabsorption and complete filterability of PAH)?

$$C_{In} = \frac{U_{In}V}{P_{In}}$$

$$= \frac{100 \text{ mg/100 ml}}{1 \text{ mg/100 ml}} \times 1.4 \text{ liters/day}$$

$$= 140 \text{ liters/day}$$

$$C_{urea} = \frac{U_{urea}V}{P_{urea}}$$

$$= \frac{220 \text{ mmol/liter}}{5 \text{ mmol/liter}} \times 1.4 \text{ liters/day}$$

$$= 61.6 \text{ liters/day}$$

$$C_{PAH} = \frac{U_{PAH}V}{P_{PAH}}$$

$$= \frac{700 \text{ mg/ml} \times 1.4 \text{ liters/day}}{2 \text{ mg/ml}}$$

$$= 490 \text{ liters/day}$$

ERPF = 490 liters/day

ERBF $= 817$ liters/day

$$\begin{aligned}\text{Reabsorbed} \atop \text{urea} &= \text{filtered urea}\\ &\quad - \text{excreted urea}\\ &= (140 \text{ liters/day}\\ &\quad \times 5 \text{ mmol/liter}) -\\ &\quad (220 \text{ mmol/liter}\\ &\quad \times 1.4 \text{ liters/day})\\ &= 392 \text{ mmol/day}\end{aligned}$$

$$\begin{aligned}\text{PAH secreted} &= \text{PAH excreted}\\ &\quad - \text{PAH filtered}\\ &= (700 \text{ mg/ml}\\ &\quad \times 1.4 \text{ liters/day})\\ &\quad - (2 \text{ mg/ml}\\ &\quad \times 140 \text{ liters/day})\\ &= 980 \text{ gm/day}\\ &\quad - 280 \text{ gm/day}\\ &= 700 \text{ gm/day}\end{aligned}$$

p32 PAH Clearance changes c̄ Plasma Conc.

8 An increase in the plasma concentration of inulin causes which of the following in the renal clearance of inulin:

  a Increase
  b Decrease
  c No change

c. $C_{In} = U_{In}V/P_{In}$. When P_{In} increases, there is no change in C_{In} because U_{In} rises an identical amount. In other words, the mass of inulin filtered and excreted increases but the volume of plasma supplying this inulin, i.e., completely cleared of inulin, is unaltered.

9 The clearance of substance A is less than that simultaneously determined for inulin. Give three possible explanations.

(1) Substance A is, itself, a large molecule poorly filtered at the glomerulus.
(2) Substance A is bound, at least in part, to plasma protein.
(3) Substance A is reabsorbed.

10 List in order of decreasing renal clearance the following substances:

  Glucose
  Urea
  Sodium
  Inulin

PAH
Creatinine
Inulin
Urea

Creatinine
PAH
Phosphate

Phosphate
Sodium
Glucose

11 If 50 percent of the nephrons were destroyed, which of the following compounds would be likely to show an increased blood concentration?

  a Urea
  b Creatinine
  c Uric acid
  d Most amino acids
  e Glucose
  f Purines

a, b, c. These waste products are all normally excreted in large amounts; a decreased GFR would cause their plasma concentrations to increase until filtered load was increased enough to reestablish normal excretion. In contrast, the reabsorption T_m's for glucose, amino acids, purines, and many other organic compounds which are not waste products are usually so high as to prevent significant excretion. Accordingly, their plasma concentrations are virtually independent of renal function; i.e., the kidneys do not participate in the setting of their plasma concentrations.

12 A month after 80 percent of the nephrons are destroyed, what will the blood urea concentration be, assuming it was 5 mmol/liter before the disease occurred.

  a 25 mmol/liter
  b 5 mmol/liter
  c 6 mmol/liter
  d Continuously rising
  e Not calculable unless it is assumed that the patient's protein intake did not change as a result of the disease

e. If one assumes a constant protein intake, then 25 mmol/liter would have been the correct answer, since total filtered urea could be restored to normal at this point $[25(0.2 \times 180) = 5 \times 180]$. However, had protein intake been reduced by 50 percent, then plasma urea would stabilize at 12.5 mmol/liter since only 50 percent as much urea would be produced.

13 During a dog experiment, a clamp around the renal artery is partially tightened so as to reduce renal arterial pressure from a mean of 120 mmHg to 80 mmHg. How much do you predict RBF will change?

  a 33-percent decrease
  b Zero

c. Autoregulation prevents the RBF from decreasing in direct proportion to mean arterial pressure, but autoregulation is not 100 percent.

c   5 to 10-percent decrease
d   33-percent increase

14 A patient suffers a hemorrhage which drops his mean arterial pressure by 25 percent. What do you predict happens to his GFR and RBF?
a   Almost no change
b   A fairly large decrease, RBF > GFR

b. If you answered "a," you probably assumed that autoregulation would prevent any significant change. This is wrong because the drop in pressure reflexly stimulates increased sympathetic tone to the kidney. (See text for the reason the GFR change is less than the RBF change.)

15 In the steady state, what is the amount of sodium chloride excreted daily in the urine by a normal person ingesting 12 gm of sodium chloride per day?
a   12 gm/day
b   Less than 12 gm/day

b. Urinary excretion in the steady state must be less than ingested sodium chloride by an amount equal to that lost in the sweat and feces. This is normally quite small, less than 1 gm/day, so that urine excretion in this case equals approximately 11 g/day.

16 A person's plasma sodium concentration is 144 mmol/liter, and his inulin clearance is 120 ml/min. His urine volume is 36 ml in 30 min, and the urine sodium concentration is 200 mmol/liter. <u>What percent of filtered sodium is</u> <u>he excreting?</u>

1.4%

Filtered Na^+ = 144 mmol/liter
$\times$ 0.12 liter/min
= 17.28 mmol/min

Excreted Na^+ = 0.036 liter/ 30 min $\times$ 200 mmol/liter
= 0.24 mmol/min

$$\% \frac{\text{Excreted}}{\text{Filtered}} = \frac{0.24}{17.28}$$
$$\times 100 = 1.4\%$$

17 Complete inhibition of active sodium reabsorption would cause an increase in the excretion of which of the following substances?
a   Water
b   Urea
c   Chloride
d   Glucose

a, b, c. Water and chloride (in most of the tubule) are reabsorbed passively as a result of electrochemical gradients generated by active sodium reabsorption. Urea is reabsorbed passively as a result of concentration gradients established by water reabsorption and is thus reabsorbed indirectly by sodium reabsorption. Glucose has its own active-transport system.

18 In chronic renal disease plasma urea may become markedly elevated. Under such circumstances urea will act as an osmotic diuretic. What does this do to sodium, chloride, and water excretion?

Sodium, chloride, and water excretion will all increase.

19 Normally there are no *passive* fluxes of sodium into or out of the proximal tubule. True or false?

False. There are very large passive fluxes in both directions. However, there is no *net* flux because of the absence of a significant electrochemical gradient for sodium.

20 a Complete inhibition of active chloride transport by the ascending loop of Henle would virtually eliminate the ability to excrete a concentrated urine. True or false?

b Increasing the passive permeability of the ascending loop to chloride would reduce the maximal concentrating ability of the kidney. True or false?

c Active reabsorption of sodium by the descending loop is a component of the countercurrent multiplier system. True or false?

(*a*) True.
(*b*) True. The gradient between ascending loop and interstitium at any *horizontal* level would be decreased; therefore the gradient from top to bottom would be decreased.
(*c*) False. There is no reabsorption of sodium (or chloride) by the descending loop.

21 True or false questions.
  a Net reabsorption of sodium occurs in the ascending loop of Henle.
  b Net reabsorption of water occurs in the descending loop.
  c Net reabsorption of water occurs in the collecting ducts.
  d Net bulk flow of interstitial fluid into the vasa recta occurs.

All are true. The last may have given you trouble. The fact is that the vasa recta act as countercurrent exchangers to eliminate net overall *diffusion* of sodium and water into or out of the vasa recta by balancing any net movements in the descending vessels with opposite ones in the ascending. Thus, net diffusional movements are minimal, but normal capillary *bulk flow* must still be occurring, or otherwise the sodium and water reabsorbed from the loops of Henle and collecting duct would not be carried away.

22 In an experiment a dog's rate of glomerular filtration of sodium is found to be 15 mmol/min.

  a How much sodium do you predict remains in the tubule at the end of the proximal tubule?

  b His GFR is suddenly increased by 33 percent. How much sodium now is left at the end of the proximal tubule?

(*a*) 5 mmol/min. Approximately two-thirds of filtered sodium is reabsorbed by the proximal tubule. (*b*) 6.6 mmol/min. Filtered sodium rises from 15 to 20 mmol/min. Glomerulotubular balance maintains sodium reabsorption at approximately two-thirds of the filtered load. If no glomerulotubular balance had occurred, then the proximal would have continued to reabsorb 10 mmol/min, and $20 - 10 = 10$ mmol/min (rather than 6.6) would remain at the end of the proximal. This should reinforce the damping effect glomerulotubular balance exerts on the ability of GFR changes, per se, to influence sodium excretion greatly.

23 Normally aldosterone controls the reabsorption of approximately 33 gm of sodium chloride per day. If a patient loses 100 percent of his adrenal function, will he excrete 33 gm of sodium chloride per day indefinitely?

No. As soon as he starts to become sodium-deficient as a result of the increased sodium excretion, the usual sodium-retaining reflexes will be set into motion. They will, of course, be unable to raise aldosterone secretion, but they will lower GFR and alter third factor so as to at least partially compensate for the decreased aldosterone-dependent sodium reabsorption.

24 What happens to sodium excretion during quiet standing?

It decreases. Because of venous pooling of blood and increased filtration of fluid across the leg capillaries, quiet standing causes an effective decrease in plasma volume, which triggers all the described inputs leading to decreased sodium excretion (decreased GFR and increased tubular reabsorption).

25 A patient has just suffered a severe hemorrhage and his plasma

No. It will probably be above normal because of an increased fil-

protein concentration is normal (not enough time has elapsed for interstitial fluid to move into the plasma). Does this mean that his peritubular-capillary colloid osmotic pressure is also normal?

26 A patient with severe liver disease has a plasma albumin of 2.5 gm/100 ml. He retains virtually all the sodium he eats (i.e., his urinary excretion of sodium is close to zero) and is becoming edematous. What is the stimulus for renal sodium retention in this case, since total extracellular volume is clearly greater than normal?

tration fraction secondary to sympathetically mediated renal arteriolar constriction.

Because of the low plasma albumin, his *plasma volume is decreased* as a result of the abnormal balance of forces across the capillaries of his body. This decreased plasma volume initiated sodium-retaining reflexes just as if the plasma volume had been decreased by diarrhea, a burn, etc. The retained fluid does not restore the plasma volume to normal, however, but merely filters into the interstitium, where it increases the edema. Interestingly, tubular sodium reabsorption is increased in this state despite the fact that peritubular-capillary protein concentration, a component of so-called third-factor, must be lower than normal, which should reduce tubular sodium reabsorption. A reflexly increased aldosterone level is certainly important in stimulating sodium reabsorption and overriding this effect of the low protein. Changes in renal hemodynamics and in the postulated natriuretic hormone may also be important.

27 A patient is suffering from primary hyperaldosteronism, i.e., increased secretion of aldosterone, usually caused by an aldosterone-producing adrenal tumor. Is his plasma renin concentration higher or lower than normal?

Lower. The increased aldosterone causes positive sodium balance which reflexly inhibits renin secretion. Thus one observes a high plasma aldosterone and a low plasma renin—a strong tip-off as to the presence of the disease, since in almost all other situations renin and aldosterone change in the same direction (because renin-angiotensin is the major control of aldosterone secretion).

28 Any agent which increases sodium and water excretion is called a diuretic, even though natriuretic is probably a better term. List possible mechanisms of actions of these drugs.

(1) Increase GFR either by raising blood pressure or by dilating renal afferent arterioles.
(2) The above hemodynamic changes would also inhibit sodium reabsorption by increasing peritubular-capillary hydrostatic pressure and/or reducing peritubular-capillary oncotic pressure (because of decreased filtration fraction).
(3) Directly inhibit the active-transport system for sodium, e.g., by blocking its energy supply, or for chloride (in the loop).
(4) Inhibit secretion of renin or aldosterone.
(5) Block action of aldosterone.
(6) Act as an osmotic diuretic by its osmotic contribution (mannitol, for example).
(7) Inhibit active secretory system for hydrogen (e.g., by blocking carbonic anhydrase). (You will not know this now, but will by the end of the book.)
This list is by no means exhaustive, but does include the major clinically useful types of diuretics.

29 A normal subject loses 2 liters of isotonic salt solution because of diarrhea. He simultaneously drinks 2 liters of pure water. What happens to:
  a Extracellular-fluid volume
  b Body-fluid osmolarity
  c Renin and aldosterone secretion
  d ADH secretion

(*a*) and (*b*) Extracellular volume and osmolarity both decrease. The entire 2 liters of solution was lost from the extracellular compartment, since it was isotonic (therefore osmolarity did not change and no water moved into or out of cells). The 2 liters of ingested pure water is distributed throughout the body water, only about one-third remaining in the extracellular fluid. Moreover, the addition of pure water lowers the osmolarity.

(*c*) Increases, because of reflexes induced by the decreased extracellular volume.

(*d*) Cannot predict. The decreased extracellular volume reflexly stimulates ADH secretion, but the reduced osmolarity should inhibit it via the hypothalamic osmoreceptors.

30 A person excretes 2 liters of urine having an osmolarity of 600 mOsm/liter. As a result, does his body-fluid osmolarity *increase* or *decrease?* The change would be identical to that produced by *adding or subtracting* (*?*) *how many* liters of pure water to/from his body?

Decrease, adding, 2 liters. He has excreted 2 liters × 600 mOsm/liter = 1,200 mOsm total solute and 2 liters water. Two liters of normal body fluids contain 2 liters × 300 mOsm/liter = 600 mOsm solutes. Accordingly, he has excreted 1,200 − 600 = 600 mOsm pure solute beyond that needed for isotonicity. This will reduce the body-fluid osmolarity by an amount equivalent to that produced by adding 2 liters pure water.

31 A person excreted 3 liters of urine having an osmolarity of 150 mOsm/liter. As a result, does his body-fluid osmolarity *increase* or *decrease?* The change is identical to that produced by *adding or subtracting* (*?*) *how many* liters pure water to/from the body?

Increase, subtracting, 1.5 liters. He has excreted 3 liters × 150 mOsm/liter = 450 mOsm total solute and 3 liters water. This amount of solute is contained in 450 mOsm ÷ 300 mOsm/liter = 1.5 liters normal body fluid. Therefore he has excreted 3 liters − 1.5 liters = 1.5 liters pure water from the body, thereby raising its osmolarity.

32 What are the major renal sites of action of the following hormones?
   Aldosterone
   ADH
   Renin
   Epinephrine

Aldosterone: Distal tubule and collecting duct
ADH: Distal tubule and collecting duct
Renin: No renal site of action
Epinephrine: Renal arterioles and JG apparatus

33 What are the major controls of aldosterone secretion rate? Which is most important?

(1) Angiotensin: most important
(2) ACTH
(3) Plasma sodium concentration
(4) Plasma potassium concentration

34 What are the major controls of renin secretion?

(1) Afferent arteriolar pressure (intrarenal baroreceptor theory)
(2) Sodium load to the macula densa
(3) Activity of renal sympathetic nerves
(4) Angiotensin

35 What are the major controls of ADH secretion:

(1) Body-fluid osmolarity via hypothalamic osmoreceptors
(2) Plasma volume (specifically left atrial pressure via baroreceptors)

36 Control of potassium excretion is achieved mainly by regulating the rate of:
  a Potassium filtration
  b Potassium reabsorption
  c Potassium secretion

c

37 A patient has a tumor in the adrenal which continuously secretes large quantities of aldosterone (primary hyperaldosteronism). Is his rate of potassium excretion normal, high, or low?

High. The increased aldosterone stimulates potassium secretion and, thereby, excretion. Interestingly, there is no potassium escape similar to the sodium escape from aldosterone.

38 A person in previously normal potassium balance maintains neurotic hyperventilation for several days. During this period what happens to his potassium balance?

It becomes negative. The hyperventilation causes alkalosis, which in turn induces increased secretion of potassium (probably due to an alkalosis-induced elevation of renal tubular cell potassium concentration).

39 A patient with severe congestive heart failure is secreting large quantities of aldosterone. Is his rate of potassium excretion normal, high, or low?

Relatively normal. This is a difficult question. You may well have answered "high" assuming that the increased aldosterone would stimulate potassium secretion. However, this effect is more than balanced by the fact that the patient is putting out almost no sodium. Recall that potassium secretion is greatly impaired when the amount of fluid flowing through the distal tubule is reduced. This explains why patients with the diseases of secondary hyperaldosteronism do not lose large quantities of potassium; whereas patients with primary hyperaldosteronism do. (Recall that the latter show escape, i.e., resumption of normal sodium excretion and distal-tubular flow despite elevated aldosterone.)

40 A patient is observed to excrete 2 liters of alkaline (pH = 7.6) urine having a bicarbonate concentration of 28 mmol/liter. His rate of titratable acid excretion is:

  a 56 mmol
  b Negative
  c Cannot tell without data for ammonium

b. If his urine has a pH greater than 7.4, then clearly there is no titratable acid (t.a.) excreted; indeed, there is negative t.a. excretion. Ammonium does not contribute to t.a. and may be ignored in the calculation of t.a.

41 The following data are obtained for a subject:

$$C_{In} = 170 \text{ liters/day}$$
$$P_{HCO_3^-} = 25 \text{ mmol/liter}$$
$$U_{HCO_3^-} = 0$$
Urine pH = 5.8
Titratable acid = 26 mmol/day
Urine NH_4^+ = 48 mmol/day

  a Calculate: Total hydrogen ion secreted
  b New bicarbonate added to the blood, i.e., acid excreted

(*a*) 4,324 mmol/day. (Sum of HCO_3^- reabsorbed, t.a. excreted, and NH_4^+ excreted.)
(*b*) 74 mmol/day. (Sum of t.a. and NH_4^+.)

42 Which values could you predict are those for a patient with primary hyperaldosteronism?

	Urine pH	Plasma pH
a	6.9	7.55
b	8.2	7.55
c	4.8	7.30

a. A very difficult bonus question. This patient secretes excessive amounts of aldosterone, which induces potassium deficiency (because of increased renal potassium secretion). The potassium deficiency then induces inappropriately large renal hydrogen-ion secretion, thereby producing a metabolic alkalosis. Note that the urine is still acid, i.e., the kidneys cannot compensate because of the potassium deficiency.

43 If renal tubular carbonic anhydrase were completely inhibited, you would expect increased excretion of which of the following?
  a Sodium
  b Water
  c Chloride
  d Bicarbonate
  e Ammonium

a, b, and d. The basic defect will be decreased acid secretion; see text for explanation. If anything, chloride excretion will decrease because of the reciprocal relationship between bicarbonate and chloride reabsorption. Ammonium excretion will be close to nil because the alkalinity of the tubular fluid minimizes diffusion trapping of ammonia.

44 Match the top column with the bottom column. ("Increased" or "decreased" is with reference to normal.)
  a Diabetic ketoacidosis
  b Hypoventilation
  c Excessive ingestion of sodium bicarbonate

  1. Increased plasma pH, increased plasma bicarbonate, alkaline urine
  2. Decreased plasma pH, decreased plasma bicarbonate, acidic urine
  3. Decreased plasma pH, increased plasma bicarbonate, acidic urine

(a) 2
(b) 3
(c) 1

45 A patient has vomited several liters of gastric juice containing large quantities of hydrochloric acid and potassium. His urine is consistently acid, and his plasma pH alkaline. Name two reasons for the failure of the kidneys to compensate for the alkalosis.

(1) He is volume-contracted because of the chloride and water loss.
(2) He is potassium deficient.
  Both (1) and (2) cause inappropriately elevated hydrogen-ion secretion.

46 Which of the following would you expect to find in a patient suffering from primary hypersecretion of parathyroid hormone?

    a Increased plasma calcium
    b Decreased plasma phosphate
    c Increased urine calcium
    d Increased tubular reabsorption of calcium
    e Increased urine phosphate
    f Increased plasma calcitonin

All are correct. c and d are not mutually exclusive because of the marked increase in filtered calcium. Calcitonin is reflexly increased by the increased plasma calcium.

Suggested Readings

GENERAL

Berliner, R. W., and J. Orloff (eds.): "Handbook of Renal Physiology," sec. 8, American Physiological Society, Wash., D.C., 1973.

Pitts, R. F.: "Physiology of the Kidney and Body Fluids," 3d ed., Year Book, Chicago, 1974.

Rouiller, C., and A. F. Muller (eds.): "The Kidney," Academic, New York, 1969–1971. (4 vols.)

Wesson, L. G., Jr.: "Physiology of the Human Kidney," Grune & Stratton, New York, 1969.

The book by Pitts is quite readable and is the best place to begin when one wishes to explore an area in greater depth. In contrast to this book, those by Wesson, Rouiller and Muller, and Berliner and Orloff are large reference books. The "Handbook" is, without question, the single most valuable reference source for renal physiology. Its articles are comprehensive and authoritative (as well as long and difficult), and their bibliographies provide a systematic entry to the original literature.

For the student who wishes to pursue continuing developments in renal physiology, the best journals to peruse are: *American Journal of Physiology, Circulation Research, Journal of Clinical Investigation, Kidney International, Pflüegers Archiv (European Journal of Physiology)*. The *New England Journal of Medicine* also frequently publishes excellent review articles on renal physiology.

RESEARCH TECHNIQUES

Burg, M., and J. Orloff: Perfusion of Isolated Renal Tubules, in R. W. Berliner and J. Orloff (eds.), "Handbook of Renal Physiology," sec. 8, American Physiological Society, Wash., D.C., 1973.

Gottschalk, C. W., and W. E. Lassiter: Micropuncture Methodology, in R. W. Berliner and J. Orloff (eds.), "Handbook of Renal Physiology," sec. 8, American Physiological Society, Wash., D.C., 1973.

Levinsky, N. G., and M. Levy: Clearance Techniques, in R. W. Berliner and J. Orloff (eds.), "Handbook of Renal Physiology," sec. 8, American Physiological Society, Wash., D.C., 1973.

Malvin, R. L., and W. S. Wilde: Stop-flow Technique, in R. W. Berliner and J. Orloff (eds.), "Handbook of Renal Physiology," sec. 8, American Physiological Society, Wash., D.C., 1973.

CHAP. 1

Barger, A. C., and J. A. Herd: Renal Vascular Anatomy and Distribution of Blood Flow, in R. W. Berliner and J. Orloff (eds.), "Handbook of Renal Physiology," sec. 8, American Physiological Society, Wash., D.C., 1973.

Dalton, A. J., and F. Hagenau (eds.): "Ultrastructure of the Kidney," Academic, New York, 1967.

Oliver, J.: "Nephrons and Kidneys: A Quantitative Study of Developmental and Evolutionary Mammalian Architectonics," Harper & Row, New York, 1968.

Rouiller, C., and A. F. Muller (eds.): "The Kidney," vol. 1, Academic, New York, 1969.

CHAP. 2

Deen, W. M., C. R. Robertson, and B. M. Brenner: Glomerular Ultrafiltration, *Fed. Proc.*, **33**:14 (1974). The most concise review of glomerular pressures and the dependence of GFR on RBF.

Kassirer, J. P.: Clinical Evaluation of Kidney Function—Tubular Function, *New Eng. J. Med.*, **285**:499 (1971).

Latta, H.: The Glomerular Capillary Wall, *J. Ultrastruct. Res.* **32**:526 (1970).

Maddox, D. A., W. M. Deen, and B. M. Brenner: Dynamics of Glomerular Ultrafiltration: VI. Studies in the Primate, *Kidney Int.*, **5**:271 (1974).

Pappenheimer, J. R.: Passage of Molecules through Capillary Walls, *Physiol.*

Rev., **33:**387 (1953). A discussion of the basic concepts and principles of ultrafiltration.

Pitts, R. F.: "Physiology of the Kidney and Body Fluids," 3d ed., chaps. 6 and
8, Year Book, Chicago, 1974. General descriptions of tubular reabsorption
and secretion. This is also a good source of information on the transport
systems for specific substances (glucose, phosphate, etc.).

Renkin, E. M., and J. Gilmore: Glomerular Filtration, in R. W. Berliner and J.
Orloff (eds.), "Handbook of Renal Physiology," sec. 8, American Physiological Society, Wash., D.C., 1973.

Renkin, E. M., and R. R. Robinson: Glomerular Filtration, *New Eng. J. Med.,*
290:785 (1974).

CHAP. 3

Kassirer, J. P.: Clinical Evaluation of Kidney Function—Glomerular Function,
New Eng. J. Med., **285:**385 (1971).

Levinsky, N. G., and M. Levy: Clearance Techniques, in R. W. Berliner and J.
Orloff (eds.), "Handbook of Renal Physiology," sec. 8, American Physiological Society, Wash., D.C., 1973.

Smith, H. W.: "Principles of Renal Physiology," chap. 3–6, Oxford, N.Y., 1956.

CHAP. 4

Barger, A. C., and J. A. Herd: Renal Vascular Anatomy and Distribution of
Blood Flow, in R. W. Berliner and J. Orloff (eds.), "Handbook of Renal
Physiology," sec. 8, American Physiological Society, Wash., D.C., 1973.

Barger, A. C., and J. A. Herd: The Renal Circulation, *New Eng. J. Med.,*
284:482 (1971).

Deen, W. M., C. R. Robertson, and B. M. Brenner: Glomerular Ultrafiltration,
Fed. Proc., **33**(1):14 (1974). Helps explain why autoregulation of RBF automatically yields autoregulation of GFR as well.

Johnson, P. C. (ed.): Autoregulation of Blood Flow, *Circ. Res.,* vol. 15, supple-
ment I, 1964, p. 103–200.

McGiff, J. C., K. Crowshaw, and H. D. Itskovitz: Prostaglandins and Renal
Function, *Fed. Proc.,* **33**(1):39 (1974). This should reinforce the fact that a
variety of humoral agents may influence renal hemodynamics (and renal
function, in general).

Selkurt, E. E.: The Renal Circulation, in W. I. Hamilton and P. Dow, "Handbook of Physiology," sec. 2, vol. II, American Physiological Society,
Wash., D.C., 1963.

Wright, Fred S.: Intrarenal Regulation of Glomerular Filtration Rate, *New Eng.
J. Med.,* **291:**135 (1974). An attempt to explain GFR autoregulation in
terms of a glomerulartubular feedback.

CHAP. 5

Burg, M. B., and J. Orloff: Perfusion of Isolated Renal Tubules, in R. W.
Berliner and J. Orloff (eds.), "Handbook of Renal Physiology," sec. 8,
American Physiological Society, Wash., D.C., 1973.

Giebisch, G.: Coupled Ion and Fluid Transport in the Kidney, *New Eng. J. Med.*, **287:**913 (1972).

Giebisch, G.: Some Recent Developments in Renal Electrolyte Transport, in L. G. Wesson and G. M. Fanelli, Jr. (eds.), "Recent Advances in Renal Physiology and Pharmacology," University Park Press, Baltimore, 1974.

Giebisch, G., and E. Windhager: Electrolyte Transport Across Renal Tubular Membranes, in R. W. Berliner and J. Orloff (eds.), "Handbook of Renal Physiology," sec. 8, American Physiological Society, Wash., D.C., 1973.

Kokko, J. P.: Membrane Characteristics Governing Salt and Water Transport in the Loop of Henle, *Fed. Proc.*, **33**(1):25 (1974). An excellent discussion of several of the complexities we glossed over: role of urea, distinction between thin and thick ascending loop, etc.

Schmidt-Nielsen, B. (ed.): "Urea and the Kidney," Excerpta Medica Foundation, Amsterdam, 1970. Role of urea in renal concentrating mechanisms.

Windhager, E. E., and G. Giebisch: Electrophysiology of the Nephron, *Physiol. Rev.*, **45:**214, 1965.

Wirz, H., and R. Dirix: Urinary Concentration and Dilution, in R. W. Berliner and J. Orloff (eds.), "Handbook of Renal Physiology," sec. 8, American Physiological Society, Wash., D.C., 1973.

Wirz, H., and F. Spinelli (eds.): "Recent Advances in Renal Physiology," Karger, Basel, 1972. A symposium with many articles concerning most controversial aspects of the mechanisms of fluid reabsorption: role of bulk flow, role of peritubular pressures, nature of chloride transport, role of ADH, etc.

CHAP. 6

Anderson, B.: "Thirst—and Brain Control of Water Balance, *Amer. Sci.*, **59:**408 (1971).

Brenner, B. M., and J. L. Troy: "Postglomerular Vascular Protein Concentration: Evidence for a Causal Role in Governing Fluid Reabsorption and Glomerulotubular Balance by the Renal Proximal Tubule, *J. Clin. Invest*, **50:**336 (1971).

Davis, J. O.: The Control of Renin Release, *Amer. J. Med.*, **55:**333 (1973).

Denton, D. A.: Salt Appetite, in C. F. Code and W. Heidel (eds.), "Handbook of Physiology," sec. 6, vol. I, American Physiological Society, 1967.

De Wardener, H. E.: The Control of Sodium Excretion, in R. W. Berliner and J. Orloff (eds.), "Handbook of Renal Physiology," sec. 8, American Physiological Society, Wash., D.C., 1973.

Earley, L. E., and T. M. Daugharty: Sodium Metabolism, *New Eng. J. Med.*, **281:**72 (1969).

Earley, L. E., and R. W. Schrier: Intrarenal Control of Sodium Excretion by Hemodynamic and Physical Factors, in R. W. Berliner and J. Orloff (eds.), "Handbook of Renal Physiology," sec. 8, American Physiological Society, Wash., D.C., 1973.

Gauer, D. H., and J. P. Henry: Circulatory Basis of Fluid Volume Control, *Physiol. Rev.*, **43:**423 (1963).

Handler, J. S., and J. Orloff: The Mechanism of Action of Antidiuretic Hormone, in R. W. Berliner and J. Orloff (eds.), "Handbook of Renal Physiology," sec. 8, American Physiological Society, Wash., D.C., 1973.

Laragh, J. H., and J. E. Sealey: The Renin-Angiotensin-Aldosterone Hormonal System and Regulation of Sodium, Potassium, and Blood Pressure Homeostasis, in R. W. Berliner and J. Orloff (eds.), "Handbook of Renal Physiology," sec. 8, American Physiological Society, Wash., D.C., 1973.

Oparil, S., and E. Haber: The Renin-Angiotensin System, *New Eng. J. Med.,* **291:**389 (1974).

Schrier, R. W., and H. E. de Wardener: Tubular Reabsorption of Sodium Ion: Influence of Factors Other Than Aldosterone and Glomerular Filtration Rate, *New Eng. J. Med.,* **285:**1231 (1971). The most extensive review of third factor.

Schwartz, I. L., and W. B. Schwarz (eds.), Symposium on Antidiuretic Hormones, *Amer. J. Med.,* **42:**651 (1967).

Sharp, G. W. G., and A. Leaf: Effects of Aldosterone and Its Mechanism of Action on Sodium Transport, in R. W. Berliner and J. Orloff (eds.), "Handbook of Renal Physiology," sec. 8, American Physiological Society, Wash., D.C., 1973.

Smith, H. W.: Salt and Water Volume Receptors, *Amer. J. Med.,* **23:**623 (1957).

Stein, J. H., and H. J. Reineck: The Role of the Collecting Duct in the Regulation of Excretion of Sodium and Other Electrolytes, *Kidney Int.,* **6:**1 (1974).

Vander, A. J.: Control of Renin Release, *Physiol. Rev.,* **47:**359, 1967.

Windhager, E. E.: Some Aspects of Proximal Tubular Salt Reabsorption, *Fed. Proc.,* **33**(1):21 (1974). A concise review of the role of peritubular pressures in sodium reabsorption.

CHAP. 7

Brenner, B. M., and R. W. Berliner: Transport of Potassium, in R. W. Berliner and J. Orloff (eds.), "Handbook of Renal Physiology," sec. 8, American Physiological Society, Wash., D.C., 1973.

Giebisch, G.: Coupled Ion and Fluid Transport in the Kidney, *New Eng. J. Med.,* **287:**913 (1972).

Giebisch, G.: Renal Potassium Excretion, in C. Rouiller and A. F. Muller (eds.), "The Kidney," vol. 3, Academic, New York, 1971.

Stein, J. H., and H. J. Reineck: The Role of the Collecting Duct in the Regulation and Excretion of Sodium and Other Electrolytes, *Kidney Int.,* **6:**1 (1974).

CHAP. 8

Giebisch, G.: Coupled Ion and Fluid Transport in the Kidney, *New Eng. J. Med.,* **287:**913 (1972).

Malnic, G., and G. Giebisch: Mechanism of Renal Hydrogen Ion Secretion, *Kidney Int.,* **1:**280 (1972).

Pitts, R. F.: Control of Renal Production of Ammonia, *Kidney Int.,* **1:**297 (1972).

Pitts, R. F.: Production and Excretion of Ammonia in Relation to Acid-Base Regulation, in R. W. Berliner and J. Orloff (eds.), "Handbook of Renal Physiology," sec. 8, American Physiological Society, Wash., D.C., 1973.

Pitts, R. F.: The Role of Ammonia Production and Excretion in Regulation of Acid-Base Balance, *New Eng. J. Med.,* **284:**32 (1971).

Rector, F. C., Jr.: Acidification of the Urine, in R. W. Berliner and J. Orloff (eds.), "Handbook of Renal Physiology," sec. 8, American Physiological Society, Wash., D.C., 1973.

Schwartz, W. B., C. Van Ypersele de Strihou, and J. P. Kassirer: Role of Anions in Metabolic Alkalosis and Potassium Deficiency, *New Eng. J. Med.,* **279:**630 (1968).

Seldin, D. W., and F. C. Rector, Jr.: The Generation and Maintenance of Metabolic Alkalosis, *Kidney Int.,* **1:**306 (1972).

CHAP. 9

Copp, D. H.: Endocrine Regulation of Calcium Metabolism, *Ann. Rev. Physiol.,* **32:**61 (1970).

DeLucca, H. F.: The Kidney as an Endocrine Organ for the Production of 1, 25-dihydroxyvitamin D_3, a Calcium-mobilizing Hormone, *New Eng. J. Med.,* **289:**359 (1973).

Massry, S. G., and J. W. Coburn: The Hormonal and Non-hormonal Control of Renal Excretion of Calcium and Magnesium, *Nephron,* **10:**66 (1973).

Rasmussen, H.: Parathyroid hormone, Calcitonin, and the Calciferols, in R. H. Williams (ed.), "Textbook of Endocrinology," 5th ed., Saunders, Philadelphia, 1974.

Walser, M.: Divalent Cations: Physicochemical State in Glomerular Filtrate and Urine and Renal Excretion, in R. W. Berliner and J. Orloff (eds.), "Handbook of Renal Physiology," sec. 8, American Physiological Society, Wash., D.C., 1973.

Index

Index

Acetoacetate:
  reabsorption of, 26
  as urinary buffer, 105
Acid excretion, 102–108
  and bicarbonate reabsorption,
    108–109
  measurement of, 111–112
Acid secretion (*see* Hydrogen ion,
    secretion of)
Acidosis:
  definition of, 100
  metabolic: causes of, 115
    renal compensation for, 115–117
  renal compensation for, 109, 112
  respiratory, renal compensation for,
    114–115
Active transport, definition of, 23
ADH (*see* Antidiuretic hormone)
Adrenal cortex, site of aldosterone
    secretion, 69
Adrenal tumor, 81
Adrenocorticotropic hormone and
    aldosterone secretion, 74
Afferent arteriole, 7
  effect of sympathetic nerves on,
    38–39
Alcohol, effect on ADH secretion, 85
Aldosterone:
  control of secretion, 74, 94–95
    by potassium, 93
  in edematous states, 80–81
  effect on potassium secretion,
    93–94
  effect on RNA, 70

effect on sodium reabsorption, 69
effects of, 94–95
and escape, 81
nonrenal effects, 69–70
site of action, 69
site of production, 69
Alkaline phosphatase, 125
Alkalosis:
  definition of, 99
  effect on potassium secretion,
    95–96, 118–119
  effect on tetany, 123
  metabolic, renal compensation for,
    116–117
  renal compensation for, 108–109,
    112
  respiratory, renal compensation for,
    115
  role of chloride, 118
  and salt depletion, 117–118
Amiloride, 97
Amino acids:
  as ammonia precursor, 106
  reabsorption by proximal tubule, 25
Ammonia:
  adaptation of synthesis, 106
  diffusion trapping of, 106–107
  passive diffusion of, 107
  pK of buffer pair, 105
  synthesis of, 106–107
  as urinary buffer, 103, 105–106
Ammonium:
  excretion of: dependence on urine
    pH, 107